MY PALEO RECIPES 2021

TASTY RECIPES FOR AVERY OCCASION

LAURA D'UBALDO

Table of Contents

Smoked Baby Back Ribs with Apple-Mustard Mop Sauce 11
Ribs 11
Sauce 11
Oven BBQ Country-Style Pork Ribs with Fresh Pineapple Slaw 14
Spicy Pork Goulash 16
Goulash 16
Cabbage 16
Italian Sausage Meatballs Marinara with Sliced Fennel and Onion Sauté 18
Meatballs 18
Marinara 18
Pork-Stuffed Zucchini Boats with Basil and Pine Nuts 20
Curried Pork and Pineapple "Noodle" Bowls with Coconut Milk and Herbs 22
Spicy Grilled Pork Patties with Tangy Cucumber Salad 24
Zucchini-Crust Pizza with Sun-Dried Tomato Pesto, Sweet Peppers, and Italian Sausage 26
Smoked Lemon-Coriander Lamb Leg with Grilled Asparagus 28
Lamb Hot Pot 30
Lamb Stew with Celery-Root Noodles 32
Frenched Lamb Chops with Pomegranate-Date Chutney 34
Chutney 34
Lamb Chops 34
Chimichurri Lamb Loin Chops with Sautéed Radicchio Slaw 36
Ancho-and-Sage-Rubbed Lamb Chops with Carrot-Sweet Potato Remoulade 38
Lamb Chops with Shallot, Mint, and Oregano Rub 40
Lamb 40
Salad 40
Garden-Stuffed Lamb Burgers with Red Pepper Coulis 42
Red Pepper Coulis 42
Burgers 42
Double-Oregano Lamb Kabobs with Tzatziki Sauce 45
Lamb Kabobs 45
Tzatziki Sauce 45

- Roast Chicken with Saffron and Lemon 47
- Spatchcocked Chicken with Jicama Slaw 49
- Chicken 49
- Slaw 49
- Roasted Chicken Hindquarters with Vodka, Carrot, and Tomato Sauce 52
- Poulet Rôti and Rutabaga Frites 54
- Triple-Mushroom Coq au Vin with Chive Mashed Rutabagas 56
- Peach-Brandy-Glazed Drumsticks 58
- Peach-Brandy Glaze 58
- Chile-Marinated Chicken with Mango-Melon Salad 60
- Chicken 60
- Salad 60
- Tandoori-Style Chicken Legs with Cucumber Raita 63
- Chicken 63
- Cucumber Raita 63
- Curried Chicken Stew with Root Vegetables, Asparagus, and Green Apple-Mint Relish 65
- Grilled Chicken Paillard Salad with Raspberries, Beets, and Roasted Almonds 67
- Broccoli Rabe-Stuffed Chicken Breasts with Fresh Tomato Sauce and Caesar Salad 69
- Grilled Chicken Shawarma Wraps with Spiced Vegetables and Pine Nut Dressing . 71
- Oven-Braised Chicken Breasts with Mushrooms, Garlic-Mashed Cauliflower, and Roasted Asparagus 73
- Thai-Style Chicken Soup 75
- Lemon and Sage Roasted Chicken with Endive 77
- Chicken with Scallions, Watercress, and Radishes 80
- Chicken Tikka Masala 82
- Ras el Hanout Chicken Thighs 85
- Star Fruit Adobo Chicken Thighs over Braised Spinach 87
- Chicken-Poblano Cabbage Tacos with Chipotle Mayo 89
- Chicken Stew with Baby Carrots and Bok Choy 91
- Cashew-Orange Chicken and Sweet Pepper Stir-Fry in Lettuce Wraps 93
- Vietnamese Coconut-Lemongrass Chicken 95
- Grilled Chicken and Apple Escarole Salad 98
- Tuscan Chicken Soup with Kale Ribbons 100
- Chicken Larb 102

Chicken Burgers with Szechwan Cashew Sauce	104
Szechwan Cashew Sauce	104
Turkish Chicken Wraps	106
Spanish Cornish Hens	108
Pistachio-Roasted Cornish Hens with Arugula, Apricot, and Fennel Salad	110
Duck Breast with Pomegranate and Jicama Salad	113
Grilled Strip Steaks with Grated Root Vegetable Hash	115
Asian Beef and Vegetable Stir-Fry	117
Cedar-Planked Filets with Asian Slather and Slaw	119
Pan-Seared Tri-Tip Steaks with Cauliflower Peperonata	122
Flat-Iron Steaks au Poivre with Mushroom-Dijon Sauce	124
Steaks	124
Sauce	124
Grilled Flat-Iron Steaks with Chipotle-Caramelized Onions and Salsa Salad	127
Steaks	127
Salsa Salad	127
Caramelized Onions	127
Grilled Ribeyes with Herbed Onion and Garlic "Butter"	130
Ribeye Salad with Grilled Beets	132
Korean-Style Short Ribs with Sautéed Ginger Cabbage	134
Beef Short Ribs with Citrus-Fennel Gremolata	137
Ribs 137	
Pan-Roasted Squash	137
Gremolata	137
Swedish-Style Beef Patties with Mustard-Dill Cucumber Salad	140
Cucumber Salad	140
Beef Patties	140
Smothered Beefburgers on Arugula with Roasted Root Vegetables	144
Grilled Beefburgers with Sesame-Crusted Tomatoes	147
Burgers on a Stick with Baba Ghanoush Dipping Sauce	149
Smoky Stuffed Sweet Peppers	151
Bison Burgers with Cabernet Onions and Arugula	153
Bison and Lamb Meat Loaf on Chard and Sweet Potatoes	156
Apple-Currant-Sauced Bison Meatballs with Zucchini Pappardelle	159
Meatballs	159

Apple-Currant Sauce ... 159
Zucchini Pappardelle ... 159
Bison-Porcini Bolognese with Roasted Garlic Spaghetti Squash ... 162
Bison Chili con Carne ... 164
Moroccan-Spiced Bison Steaks with Grilled Lemons ... 166
Herbes de Provence-Rubbed Bison Sirloin Roast ... 167
Coffee-Braised Bison Short Ribs with Tangerine Gremolata and Celery Root Mash ... 169
Marinade ... 169
Braise ... 169
Beef Bone Broth ... 172
Tunisian Spice-Rubbed Pork Shoulder with Spicy Sweet Potato Fries ... 174
Pork 174
Fries 174
Cuban Grilled Pork Shoulder ... 176
Italian Spice-Rubbed Pork Roast with Vegetables ... 179
Slow Cooker Pork Mole ... 181
Caraway-Spiced Pork and Squash Stew ... 183
Fruit-Stuffed Top Loin Roast with Brandy Sauce ... 185
Roast ... 185
Brandy Sauce ... 185
Porchetta-Style Pork Roast ... 188
Tomatillo-Braised Pork Loin ... 190
Apricot-Stuffed Pork Tenderloin ... 192
Herb-Crusted Pork Tenderloin with Crispy Garlic Oil ... 194
Indian-Spiced Pork with Coconut Pan Sauce ... 195
Pork Scaloppini with Spiced Apples and Chestnuts ... 196
Pork Fajita Stir-Fry ... 199
Pork Tenderloin with Port and Prunes ... 200
Moo Shu-Style Pork in Lettuce Cups with Quick Pickled Vegetables ... 202
Pickled Vegetables ... 202
Pork 202
Pork Chops with Macadamias, Sage, Figs, and Mashed Sweet Potatoes ... 204
Skillet-Roasted Rosemary-Lavender Pork Chops with Grapes and Toasted Walnuts ... 206

Pork Chops alla Fiorentina with Grilled Broccoli Rabe 208
Escarole-Stuffed Pork Chops 210
Pork Chops with a Dijon-Pecan Crust 213
Walnut-Crusted Pork with Blackberry Spinach Salad 214
Pork Schnitzel with Sweet-and-Sour Red Cabbage 216
Cabbage 216
Pork 216

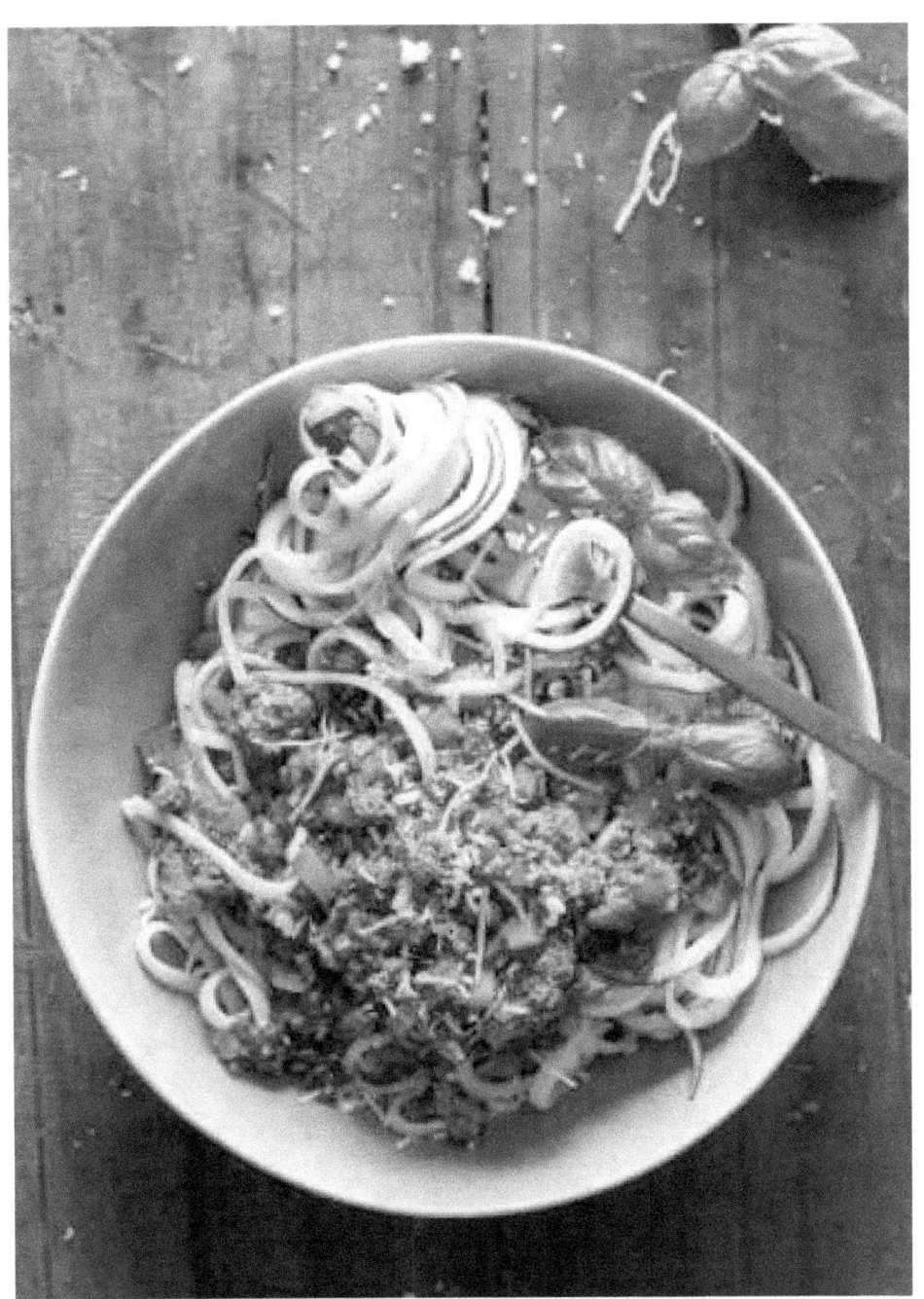

SMOKED BABY BACK RIBS WITH APPLE-MUSTARD MOP SAUCE

SOAK: 1 hour STAND: 15 minutes SMOKE: 4 hours COOK: 20 minutes MAKES: 4 servings
PHOTO

THE RICH FLAVOR AND MEATY TEXTURE OF SMOKED RIBS CALLS FOR SOMETHING COOL AND CRISP TO GO ALONG WITH IT. ALMOST ANY SLAW WILL DO, BUT THE FENNEL SLAW (SEE RECIPE AND PICTURED HERE), IS ESPECIALLY GOOD.

RIBS
- 8 to 10 apple or hickory wood chunks
- 3 to 3½ pounds pork loin baby back ribs
- ¼ cup Smoky Seasoning (see recipe)

SAUCE
- 1 medium cooking apple, peeled, cored, and thinly sliced
- ¼ cup chopped onion
- ¼ cup water
- ¼ cup cider vinegar
- 2 tablespoons Dijon-Style Mustard (see recipe)
- 2 to 3 tablespoons water

1. At least 1 hour before smoke-cooking, soak wood chunks in enough water to cover. Drain before using. Trim visible fat from ribs. If necessary, peel off the thin membrane from the back of the ribs. Place ribs in a large shallow pan. Sprinkle evenly with Smoky Seasoning; rub in with your fingers. Let stand at room temperature for 15 minutes.

2. In a smoker arrange preheated coals, drained wood chunks, and water pan according to the manufacturer's directions. Pour water into pan. Place ribs, bone sides down, on grill rack over water pan. (Or place ribs in a rib rack; place rib

rack on grill rack.) Cover and smoke for 2 hours. Maintain a temperature of about 225°F in the smoker for the duration of smoking. Add additional coals and water as needed to maintain temperature and moisture.

3. Meanwhile, for mop sauce, in a small saucepan combine apple slices, onion, and the ¼ cup water. Bring to boiling; reduce heat. Simmer, covered, for 10 to 12 minutes or until apple slices are very tender, stirring occasionally. Cool slightly; transfer undrained apple and onion to a food processor or blender. Cover and process or blend until smooth. Return puree to saucepan. Stir in vinegar and Dijon-Style Mustard. Cook over medium-low heat for 5 minutes, stirring occasionally. Add 2 to 3 tablespoons of water (or more, as needed) to make the sauce the consistency of a vinaigrette. Divide the sauce into thirds.

4. After 2 hours, brush ribs generously with one-third of the mop sauce. Cover and smoke 1 hour more. Brush again with another one-third of the mop sauce. Wrap each slab of ribs in heavy foil and place the ribs back on the smoker, layering them on top of each other if needed. Cover and smoke for 1 to 1½ hours more or until ribs are tender.*

5. Unwrap ribs and brush with the remaining one-third of the mop sauce. Cut ribs between bones to serve.

*Tip: To test tenderness of the ribs, carefully remove the foil from one of the slabs of ribs. Pick up the rib slab with tongs, holding the slab by the top one-fourth of the slab. Turn the rib slab over so the meaty side is facing down. If the ribs are tender, the slab should begin to fall apart as you pick it up. If it is not tender, wrap again in foil and continue to smoke ribs until tender.

OVEN BBQ COUNTRY-STYLE PORK RIBS WITH FRESH PINEAPPLE SLAW

PREP: 20 minutes COOK: 8 minutes BAKE: 1 hour 15 minutes MAKES: 4 servings

COUNTRY-STYLE PORK RIBS ARE MEATY, INEXPENSIVE, AND, IF TREATED THE RIGHT WAY—SUCH AS COOKED LOW AND SLOW IN A MESS OF BARBECUE SAUCE—GET MELTINGLY TENDER.

2 pounds boneless country-style pork ribs
¼ teaspoon black pepper
1 tablespoon refined coconut oil
½ cup fresh orange juice
1½ cups BBQ Sauce (see recipe)
3 cups shredded green and/or red cabbage
1 cup shredded carrots
2 cups finely chopped pineapple
⅓ cup Bright Citrus Vinaigrette (see recipe)
BBQ Sauce (see recipe) (optional)

1. Preheat oven to 350°F. Sprinkle pork with pepper. In an extra-large skillet heat coconut oil over medium-high heat. Add pork ribs; cook for 8 to 10 minutes or until browned, turning to brown evenly. Place ribs in a 3-quart rectangular baking dish.

2. For sauce, add orange juice to skillet, stirring to scrape up any browned bits. Stir in the 1½ cups BBQ Sauce. Pour sauce over ribs. Turn ribs to coat with sauce (if necessary, use a pastry brush to brush sauce over ribs). Cover baking dish tightly with aluminum foil.

3. Bake ribs for 1 hour. Remove foil and brush ribs with sauce from baking dish. Bake about 15 minutes more or until

ribs are tender and browned and sauce has thickened slightly.

4. Meanwhile, for pineapple slaw, combine cabbage, carrots, pineapple, and Bright Citrus Vinaigrette. Cover and refrigerate until serving time.

5. Serve ribs with slaw and, if desired, additional BBQ Sauce.

SPICY PORK GOULASH

PREP: 20 minutes COOK: 40 minutes MAKES: 6 servings

THIS HUNGARIAN-STYLE STEW IS SERVED ON A BED OF CRUNCHY, BARELY WILTED CABBAGE FOR A ONE-DISH MEAL. CRUSH THE CARAWAY SEEDS IN A MORTAR AND PESTLE IF YOU HAVE ONE. IF NOT, CRUSH THEM UNDER THE BROAD SIDE OF A CHEF'S KNIFE BY PRESSING DOWN ON KNIFE GENTLY WITH YOUR FIST.

GOULASH
- 1½ pounds ground pork
- 2 cups chopped red, orange, and/or yellow sweet peppers
- ¾ cup finely chopped red onion
- 1 small fresh red chile, seeded and finely chopped (see tip)
- 4 teaspoons Smoky Seasoning (see recipe)
- 1 teaspoon caraway seeds, crushed
- ¼ teaspoon ground marjoram or oregano
- 1 14-ounce can no-salt-added diced tomatoes, undrained
- 2 tablespoons red wine vinegar
- 1 tablespoon finely shredded lemon peel
- ⅓ cup snipped fresh parsley

CABBAGE
- 2 tablespoons olive oil
- 1 medium onion, sliced
- 1 small head green or red cabbage, cored and thinly sliced

1. For the goulash, in a large Dutch oven cook ground pork, sweet peppers, and onion over medium-high heat for 8 to 10 minutes or until the pork is no longer pink and vegetables are crisp-tender, stirring with a wooden spoon to break up meat. Drain off fat. Reduce heat to low; add

red chile, Smoky Seasoning, caraway seeds, and marjoram. Cover and cook for 10 minutes. Add undrained tomatoes and vinegar. Bring to boiling; reduce heat. Simmer, covered, for 20 minutes.

2. Meanwhile, for cabbage, in an extra-large skillet heat oil over medium heat. Add onion and cook until softened, about 2 minutes. Add cabbage; stir to combine. Reduce heat to low. Cook about 8 minutes or until cabbage is just tender, stirring occasionally.

3. To serve, place some of the cabbage mixture on a plate. Top with goulash and sprinkle with lemon zest and parsley.

ITALIAN SAUSAGE MEATBALLS MARINARA WITH SLICED FENNEL AND ONION SAUTÉ

PREP: 30 minutes BAKE: 30 minutes COOK: 40 minutes MAKES: 4 to 6 servings

THIS RECIPE IS A RARE EXAMPLE OF A CANNED PRODUCT WORKING AS WELL AS—IF NOT BETTER THAN—THE FRESH VERSION. UNLESS YOU HAVE TOMATOES THAT ARE VERY, VERY RIPE, YOU WILL NOT GET AS GOOD A CONSISTENCY IN A SAUCE USING FRESH TOMATOES AS YOU CAN USING CANNED TOMATOES. JUST BE SURE YOU USE A NO-SALT-ADDED PRODUCT—AND, EVEN BETTER, ORGANIC.

MEATBALLS
- 2 large eggs
- ½ cup almond meal
- 8 cloves garlic, minced
- 6 tablespoons dry white wine
- 1 tablespoon paprika
- 2 teaspoons black pepper
- 1 teaspoon fennel seeds, lightly crushed
- 1 teaspoon dried oregano, crushed
- 1 teaspoon dried thyme, crushed
- ¼ to ½ teaspoon cayenne pepper
- 1½ pounds ground pork

MARINARA
- 2 tablespoons olive oil
- 2 15-ounce cans no-salt-added crushed tomatoes or one 28-ounce can no-salt-added crushed tomatoes
- ½ cup snipped fresh basil
- 3 medium fennel bulbs, halved, cored, and thinly sliced

1 large sweet onion, halved and thinly sliced

1. Preheat oven to 375°F. Line a large rimmed baking sheet with parchment paper; set aside. In a large bowl whisk together the eggs, almond meal, 6 cloves of the minced garlic, 3 tablespoons of the wine, the paprika, 1½ teaspoons of the black pepper, the fennel seeds, oregano, thyme, and cayenne pepper. Add the pork; mix well. Shape pork mixture into 1½-inch meatballs (should have about 24 meatballs); arrange in a single layer on the prepared baking sheet. Bake about 30 minutes or until lightly browned, turning once while baking.

2. Meanwhile, for marinara sauce, in a 4- to 6-quart Dutch oven heat 1 tablespoon of the olive oil. Add the 2 remaining cloves minced garlic; cook about 1 minute or until just starting to brown. Quickly add the remaining 3 tablespoons wine, the crushed tomatoes, and the basil. Bring to boiling; reduce heat. Simmer, uncovered, for 5 minutes. Carefully stir the cooked meatballs into the marinara sauce. Cover and simmer for 25 to 30 minutes.

3. Meanwhile, in a large skillet heat the remaining 1 tablespoon olive oil over medium heat. Stir in the sliced fennel and onion. Cook for 8 to 10 minutes or until just tender and lightly browned, stirring frequently. Season with the remaining ½ teaspoon black pepper. Serve the meatballs and marinara sauce over the fennel and onion sauté.

PORK-STUFFED ZUCCHINI BOATS WITH BASIL AND PINE NUTS

PREP: 20 minutes COOK: 22 minutes BAKE: 20 minutes MAKES: 4 servings

KIDS WILL LOVE THIS FUN-TO-EAT DISH OF HOLLOWED-OUT ZUCCHINI STUFFED WITH GROUND PORK, TOMATOES, AND SWEET PEPPERS. IF YOU LIKE, STIR IN 3 TABLESPOONS OF BASIL PESTO (SEE RECIPE) IN PLACE OF THE FRESH BASIL, PARSLEY, AND PINE NUTS.

- 2 medium zucchini
- 1 tablespoon extra virgin olive oil
- 12 ounces ground pork
- ¾ cup chopped onion
- 2 cloves garlic, minced
- 1 cup chopped tomatoes
- ⅔ cup finely chopped yellow or orange sweet pepper
- 1 teaspoon fennel seeds, lightly crushed
- ½ teaspoon crushed red pepper flakes
- ¼ cup snipped fresh basil
- 3 tablespoons snipped fresh parsley
- 2 tablespoons pine nuts, toasted (see tip) and coarsely chopped
- 1 teaspoon finely shredded lemon peel

1. Preheat oven to 350°F. Halve zucchini lengthwise and carefully scrape out the center, leaving ¼-inch-thick shell. Coarsely chop the zucchini pulp and set aside. Arrange zucchini halves, cut sides up, on a foil-lined baking sheet.

2. For filling, in a large skillet heat the olive oil over medium-high heat. Add ground pork; cook until no longer pink, stirring with a wooden spoon to break up meat. Drain off fat. Reduce heat to medium. Add the reserved zucchini

pulp, onion, and garlic; cook and stir about 8 minutes or until onion is soft. Stir in the tomatoes, sweet pepper, fennel seeds, and crushed red pepper. Cook about 10 minutes or until tomatoes are soft and beginning to break down. Remove pan from heat. Stir in the basil, parsley, pine nuts, and lemon peel. Divide filling among zucchini shells, mounding slightly. Bake for 20 to 25 minutes or until zucchini shells are crisp-tender.

CURRIED PORK AND PINEAPPLE "NOODLE" BOWLS WITH COCONUT MILK AND HERBS

PREP: 30 minutes COOK: 15 minutes BAKE: 40 minutes MAKES: 4 servings PHOTO

1 large spaghetti squash

2 tablespoons refined coconut oil

1 pound ground pork

2 tablespoons finely chopped scallions

2 tablespoons fresh lime juice

1 tablespoon minced fresh ginger

6 cloves garlic, minced

1 tablespoon minced lemongrass

1 tablespoon no-salt-added Thai-style red curry powder

1 cup chopped red sweet pepper

1 cup chopped onion

½ cup julienne-cut carrot

1 baby bok choy, sliced (3 cups)

1 cup sliced fresh button mushrooms

1 or 2 Thai bird chiles, thinly sliced (see tip)

1 13.5-ounce can natural coconut milk (such as Nature's Way)

½ cup Chicken Bone Broth (see recipe) or no-salt-added chicken broth

¼ cup fresh pineapple juice

3 tablespoons unsalted no-oil-added cashew butter

1 cup cubed fresh pineapple, cubed

Lime wedges

Fresh cilantro, mint, and/or Thai basil

Chopped roasted cashews

1. Preheat oven to 400°F. Microwave spaghetti squash on high for 3 minutes. Carefully cut the squash in half lengthwise

and scrape out the seeds. Rub 1 tablespoon of the coconut oil over the cut sides of the squash. Place squash halves, cut sides down, on a baking sheet. Bake for 40 to 50 minutes or until squash can be pierced easily with a knife. Using the tines of a fork, scrape the flesh from the shells and keep warm until ready to serve.

2. Meanwhile, in a medium bowl combine the pork, scallions, lime juice, ginger, garlic, lemongrass, and curry powder; mix well. In an extra-large skillet heat the remaining 1 tablespoon of the coconut oil over medium-high heat. Add pork mixture; cook until no longer pink, stirring with a wooden spoon to break up meat. Add the sweet pepper, onion, and carrot; cook and stir about 3 minutes or until vegetables are crisp-tender. Stir in the bok choy, mushrooms, chiles, coconut milk, Chicken Bone Broth, pineapple juice, and cashew butter. Bring to boiling; reduce heat. Add pineapple; simmer, uncovered, until heated through.

3. To serve, divide the spaghetti squash among four serving bowls. Ladle the curried pork over the squash. Serve with lime wedges, herbs, and cashews.

SPICY GRILLED PORK PATTIES WITH TANGY CUCUMBER SALAD

PREP: 30 minutes GRILL: 10 minutes STAND: 10 minutes MAKES: 4 servings

THE CRUNCHY CUCUMBER SALAD FLAVORED WITH FRESH MINT IS A COOLING AND REFRESHING COMPLEMENT TO THE SPICY PORK BURGERS.

⅓ cup olive oil
¼ cup chopped fresh mint
3 tablespoons white wine vinegar
8 cloves garlic, minced
¼ teaspoon black pepper
2 medium cucumbers, very thinly sliced
1 small onion, cut into thin slivers (about ½ cup)
1¼ to 1½ pounds ground pork
¼ cup chopped fresh cilantro
1 to 2 medium fresh jalapeño or serrano chile peppers, seeded (if desired) and finely chopped (see tip)
2 medium red sweet peppers, seeded and quartered
2 teaspoons olive oil

1. In a large bowl whisk together ⅓ cup olive oil, mint, vinegar, 2 cloves minced garlic, and the black pepper. Add sliced cucumbers and onion. Toss until well coated. Cover and chill until ready to serve, stirring once or twice.

2. In a large bowl combine pork, cilantro, chile pepper, and the remaining 6 cloves minced garlic. Shape into four ¾-inch-thick patties. Brush pepper quarters lightly with the 2 teaspoons olive oil.

3. For a charcoal or gas grill, place patties and sweet pepper quarters directly over medium heat. Cover and grill until an instant-read thermometer inserted into sides of pork patties registers 160°F and pepper quarters are tender and lightly charred, turning patties and pepper quarters once halfway through grilling. Allow 10 to 12 minutes for patties and 8 to 10 minutes for the pepper quarters.

4. When pepper quarters are done, wrap them in a piece of foil to completely enclose. Let stand about 10 minutes or until cool enough to handle. Using a sharp knife, carefully peel off the pepper skins. Thinly slice pepper quarters lengthwise.

5. To serve, stir cucumber salad and spoon evenly onto four large serving plates. Add a pork patty to each plate. Pile the red pepper slices evenly on top of patties.

ZUCCHINI-CRUST PIZZA WITH SUN-DRIED TOMATO PESTO, SWEET PEPPERS, AND ITALIAN SAUSAGE

PREP: 30 minutes COOK: 15 minutes BAKE: 30 minutes MAKES: 4 servings

THIS IS KNIFE-AND-FORK PIZZA. BE SURE TO PRESS THE SAUSAGE AND PEPPERS LIGHTLY INTO THE PESTO-COATED CRUST SO THAT THE TOPPINGS ADHERE ENOUGH FOR THE PIZZA TO CUT NEATLY.

2 tablespoons olive oil

1 tablespoon finely ground almonds

1 large egg, lightly beaten

½ cup almond flour

1 tablespoon snipped fresh oregano

¼ teaspoon black pepper

3 cloves garlic, minced

3½ cups shredded zucchini (2 medium)

Italian Sausage (see recipe, below)

1 tablespoon extra virgin olive oil

1 sweet pepper (yellow, red, or half of each), seeded and cut into very thin strips

1 small onion, thinly sliced

Sun-Dried Tomato Pesto (see recipe, below)

1. Preheat oven to 425°F. Brush a 12-inch pizza pan with the 2 tablespoons olive oil. Sprinkle with ground almonds; set aside.

2. For crust, in a large bowl combine egg, almond flour, oregano, black pepper, and garlic. Place shredded zucchini in a clean towel or piece of cheesecloth. Wrap tightly

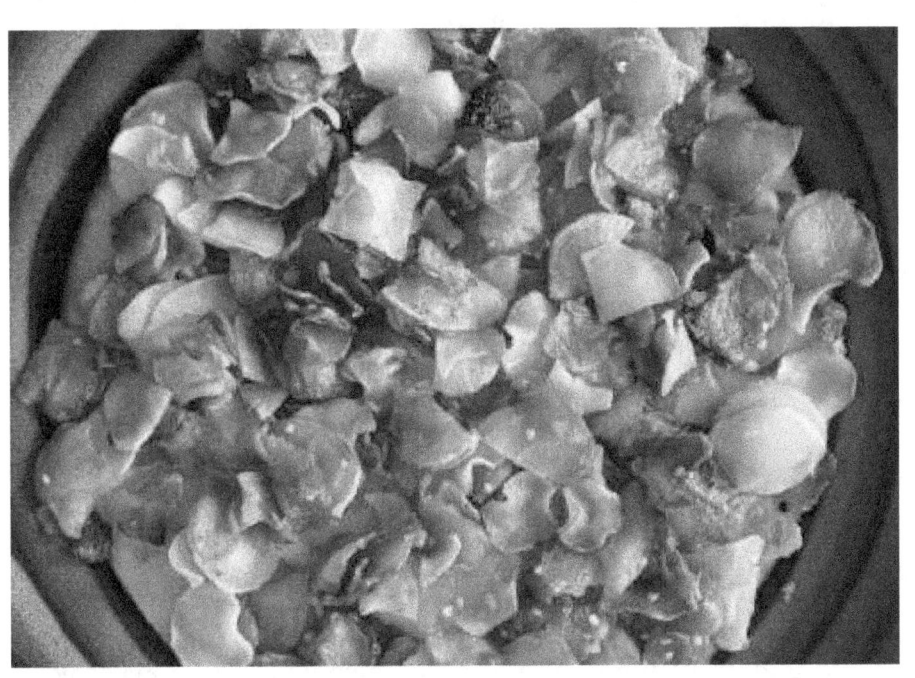

SMOKED LEMON-CORIANDER LAMB LEG WITH GRILLED ASPARAGUS

SOAK: 30 minutes PREP: 20 minutes GRILL: 45 minutes STAND: 10 minutes MAKES: 6 to 8 servings

SIMPLE BUT ELEGANT, THIS DISH FEATURES TWO INGREDIENTS THAT COME INTO THEIR OWN IN THE SPRING—LAMB AND ASPARAGUS. TOASTING THE CORIANDER SEEDS ENHANCES THE WARM, EARTHY, SLIGHTLY TANGY FLAVOR.

- 1 cup hickory wood chips
- 2 tablespoons coriander seeds
- 2 tablespoons finely shredded lemon peel
- 1½ teaspoons black pepper
- 2 tablespoons snipped fresh thyme
- 1 2- to 3-pound boneless leg of lamb
- 2 bunches fresh asparagus
- 1 tablespoon olive oil
- ¼ teaspoon black pepper
- 1 lemon, cut into quarters

1. At least 30 minutes before smoke-cooking, in a bowl soak hickory chips in enough water to cover; set aside. Meanwhile, in a small skillet toast coriander seeds over medium heat about 2 minutes or until fragrant and crackling, stirring frequently. Remove seeds from skillet; let cool. When seeds have cooled, coarsely crush in a mortar and pestle (or place seeds on a cutting board and crush them with the back of a wooden spoon). In a small bowl combine crushed coriander seeds, lemon peel, the 1½ teaspoons pepper, and thyme; set aside.

2. Remove netting from lamb roast if present. On a work surface open up the roast, fat side down. Sprinkle half of the spice mixture over meat; rub in with your fingers. Roll the roast up and tie with four to six pieces of 100%-cotton kitchen string. Sprinkle the remaining spice mixture over outside of roast, pressing lightly to adhere.

3. For a charcoal grill, arrange medium-hot coals around a drip pan. Test for medium heat above the pan. Sprinkle the drained wood chips over the coals. Place lamb roast on the grill rack over the drip pan. Cover and smoke for 40 to 50 minutes for medium (145°F). (For a gas grill, preheat grill. Reduce heat to medium. Adjust for indirect cooking. Smoke as above, except add drained wood chips according to manufacturer's directions.) Cover roast loosely with foil. Let stand for 10 minutes before slicing.

4. Meanwhile, trim woody ends from asparagus. In a large bowl toss asparagus with olive oil and the ¼ teaspoon pepper. Place asparagus around outer edges of grill, directly over the coals and perpendicular to the grill grate. Cover and grill for 5 to 6 minutes until crisp-tender. Squeeze lemon wedges over asparagus.

5. Remove string from lamb roast and thinly slice meat. Serve meat with grilled asparagus.

LAMB HOT POT

PREP: 30 minutes COOK: 2 hours 40 minutes MAKES: 4 servings

WARM UP WITH THIS SAVORY STEW ON A FALL OR WINTER NIGHT. THE STEW IS SERVED OVER A VELVETY CELERY ROOT-PARSNIP MASH FLAVORED WITH DIJON-STYLE MUSTARD, CASHEW CREAM, AND CHIVES. NOTE: CELERY ROOT IS SOMETIMES CALLED CELERIAC.

- 10 black peppercorns
- 6 sage leaves
- 3 whole allspice
- 2 2-inch strips orange peel
- 2 pounds boneless lamb shoulder
- 3 tablespoons olive oil
- 2 medium onions, coarsely chopped
- 1 14.5-ounce can no-salt-added diced tomatoes, undrained
- 1½ cups Beef Bone Broth (see recipe) or no-salt-added beef broth
- ¾ cup dry white wine
- 3 large cloves garlic, crushed and peeled
- 2 pounds celery root, peeled and cut into 1-inch cubes
- 6 medium parsnips, peeled and cut into 1-inch slices (about 2 pounds)
- 2 tablespoons olive oil
- 2 tablespoons Cashew Cream (see recipe)
- 1 tablespoon Dijon-Style Mustard (see recipe)
- ¼ cup snipped chives

1. For the bouquet garni, cut a 7-inch square of cheesecloth. Place peppercorns, sage, allspice, and orange peel in center of cheesecloth. Bring up the corners of the cheesecloth and tie securely with clean 100%-cotton kitchen string. Set aside.

2. Trim fat from lamb shoulder; cut lamb into 1-inch pieces. In a Dutch oven heat the 3 tablespoons olive oil over medium heat. Cook lamb, in batches if necessary, in hot oil until browned; remove from pan and keep warm. Add onions to pan; cook for 5 to 8 minutes or until softened and lightly browned. Add bouquet garni, undrained tomatoes, 1¼ cups of the Beef Bone Broth, wine, and garlic. Bring to boiling; reduce heat. Simmer, covered, for 2 hours, stirring occasionally. Remove and discard bouquet garni.

3. Meanwhile, for mash, place celery root and parsnips in a large stockpot; cover with water. Bring to boiling over medium-high heat; reduce heat to low. Cover and simmer gently for 30 to 40 minutes or until the vegetables are very tender when pierced with a fork. Drain; place vegetables in a food processor. Add the remaining ¼ cup Beef Bone Broth and the 2 tablespoons oil; pulse until mash is almost smooth but still has some texture, stopping once or twice to scrape down the sides. Transfer mash to a bowl. Stir in Cashew Cream, mustard, and chives.

4. To serve, divide mash among four bowls; top with Lamb Hot Pot.

LAMB STEW WITH CELERY-ROOT NOODLES

PREP: 30 minutes BAKE: 1 hour 30 minutes MAKES: 6 servings

CELERY ROOT TAKES AN ENTIRELY DIFFERENT FORM IN THIS STEW THAN IT DOES IN THE LAMB HOT POT (SEE RECIPE). A MANDOLINE SLICER IS USED TO CREATE VERY THIN STRIPS OF THE SWEET AND NUTTY-TASTING ROOT. THE "NOODLES" SIMMER IN THE STEW UNTIL THEY ARE TENDER.

2 teaspoons Lemon-Herb Seasoning (see recipe)
1½ pounds lamb stew meat, cut into 1-inch cubes
2 tablespoons olive oil
2 cups chopped onions
1 cup chopped carrots
1 cup diced turnips
1 tablespoon minced garlic (6 cloves)
2 tablespoons no-salt-added tomato paste
½ cup dry red wine
4 cups Beef Bone Broth (see recipe) or no-salt-added beef broth
1 bay leaf
2 cups 1-inch cubes butternut squash
1 cup diced eggplant
1 pound celery root, peeled
Chopped fresh parsley

1. Preheat oven to 250°F. Sprinkle Lemon-Herb Seasoning evenly over lamb. Toss gently to coat. Heat a 6- to 8-quart Dutch oven over medium-high heat. Add 1 tablespoon of the olive oil and half of the seasoned lamb to the Dutch oven. Brown meat in hot oil on all sides; transfer browned

meat to a plate and repeat with remaining lamb and olive oil. Reduce heat to medium.

2. Add onions, carrots, and turnips to pot. Cook and stir vegetables for 4 minutes; add garlic and tomato paste and cook 1 minute more. Add red wine, Beef Bone Broth, bay leaf, and reserved meat and any accumulated juices to pot. Bring mixture to a simmer. Cover and place Dutch oven in preheated oven. Bake for 1 hour. Stir in butternut squash and eggplant. Return to oven and bake for an additional 30 minutes.

3. While stew is in oven, use a mandoline to very thinly slice celery root. Cut celery root slices into ½-inch-wide strips. (You should have about 4 cups.) Stir celery root strips into stew. Simmer about 10 minutes or until tender. Remove and discard bay leaf before serving stew. Sprinkle each serving with chopped parsley.

FRENCHED LAMB CHOPS WITH POMEGRANATE-DATE CHUTNEY

PREP: 10 minutes COOK: 18 minutes COOL: 10 minutes MAKES: 4 servings

THE TERM "FRENCHED" REFERS TO A RIB BONE FROM WHICH FAT, MEAT, AND CONNECTIVE TISSUE HAVE BEEN REMOVED WITH A SHARP PARING KNIFE. IT MAKES FOR AN ATTRACTIVE PRESENTATION. ASK YOUR BUTCHER TO DO IT OR YOU CAN DO IT YOURSELF.

CHUTNEY
- ½ cup unsweetened pomegranate juice
- 1 tablespoon fresh lemon juice
- 1 shallot, peeled and thinly sliced into rings
- 1 teaspoon finely shredded orange peel
- ⅓ cup chopped Medjool dates
- ¼ teaspoon crushed red pepper
- ¼ cup pomegranate arils*
- 1 tablespoon olive oil
- 1 tablespoon chopped fresh Italian (flat-leaf) parsley

LAMB CHOPS
- 2 tablespoons olive oil
- 8 frenched lamb rib chops

1. For the chutney, in a small skillet combine pomegranate juice, lemon juice, and shallot. Bring to boiling; reduce heat. Simmer, uncovered, for 2 minutes. Add orange peel, dates, and crushed red pepper. Let stand until cool, about 10 minutes. Stir in pomegranate arils, the 1 tablespoon olive oil, and the parsley. Set aside at room temperature until serving time.

2. For the chops, in a large skillet heat the 2 tablespoons olive oil over medium heat. Working in batches, add chops to skillet and cook for 6 to 8 minutes for medium rare (145°F), turning once. Top chops with chutney.

*Note: Fresh pomegranates and their arils, or seeds, are available from October through February. If you can't find them, use unsweetened dried seeds to add crunch to the chutney.

CHIMICHURRI LAMB LOIN CHOPS WITH SAUTÉED RADICCHIO SLAW

PREP: 30 minutes MARINATE: 20 minutes COOK: 20 minutes MAKES: 4 servings

IN ARGENTINA, CHIMICHURRI IS THE MOST POPULAR CONDIMENT ACCOMPANYING THAT COUNTRY'S RENOWNED GAUCHO-STYLE GRILLED STEAK. THERE ARE LOTS OF VARIATIONS, BUT THE THICK HERB SAUCE IS USUALLY BUILT AROUND PARSLEY, CILANTRO OR OREGANO, SHALLOTS AND/OR GARLIC, CRUSHED RED PEPPER, OLIVE OIL, AND RED WINE VINEGAR. IT'S GREAT ON GRILLED STEAK BUT EQUALLY BRILLIANT ON ROASTED OR PAN-SEARED LAMB CHOPS, CHICKEN, AND PORK.

8 lamb loin chops, cut 1 inch thick
½ cup Chimichurri Sauce (see recipe)
2 tablespoons olive oil
1 sweet onion, halved and sliced
1 teaspoon cumin seeds, crushed*
1 clove garlic, minced
1 head radicchio, cored and sliced into thin ribbons
1 tablespoon balsamic vinegar

1. Place lamb chops in an extra-large bowl. Drizzle with 2 tablespoons of the Chimichurri Sauce. Using your fingers, rub the sauce over the entire surface of each chop. Let chops marinate at room temperature for 20 minutes.

2. Meanwhile, for sautéed radicchio slaw, in an extra-large skillet heat 1 tablespoon of the olive oil. Add onion, cumin seeds, and garlic; cook for 6 to 7 minutes or until onion softens, stirring frequently. Add radicchio; cook for 1 to 2

minutes or until radicchio just wilts slightly. Transfer slaw to a large bowl. Add balsamic vinegar and toss well to combine. Cover and keep warm.

3. Wipe out skillet. Add the remaining 1 tablespoon olive oil to the skillet and heat over medium-high heat. Add the lamb chops; reduce heat to medium. Cook for 9 to 11 minutes or until desired doneness, turning chops occasionally with tongs.

4. Serve chops with slaw and the remaining Chimichurri Sauce.

*Note: To crush cumin seeds, use a mortar and pestle—or place seeds on a cutting board and crush with a chef's knife.

ANCHO-AND-SAGE-RUBBED LAMB CHOPS WITH CARROT-SWEET POTATO REMOULADE

PREP: 12 minutes CHILL: 1 to 2 hours GRILL: 6 minutes MAKES: 4 servings

THERE ARE THREE TYPES OF LAMB CHOPS. THICK AND MEATY LOIN CHOPS LOOK LIKE SMALL T-BONE STEAKS. RIB CHOPS—CALLED FOR HERE—ARE CREATED BY CUTTING BETWEEN THE BONES OF A RACK OF LAMB. THEY ARE VERY TENDER AND HAVE A LONG, ATTRACTIVE BONE ON THE SIDE. THEY ARE OFTEN SERVED PAN-SEARED OR GRILLED. BUDGET-FRIENDLY SHOULDER CHOPS ARE A BIT FATTIER AND LESS TENDER THAN THE OTHER TWO TYPES. THEY ARE BEST BROWNED AND THEN BRAISED IN WINE, STOCK, AND TOMATOES—OR SOME COMBINATION OF THEM.

- 3 medium carrots, coarsely shredded
- 2 small sweet potatoes, julienne-cut* or coarsely shredded
- ½ cup Paleo Mayo (see recipe)
- 2 tablespoons fresh lemon juice
- 2 teaspoons Dijon-Style Mustard (see recipe)
- 2 tablespoons snipped fresh parsley
- ½ teaspoon black pepper
- 8 lamb rib chops, cut ½ to ¾ inch thick
- 2 tablespoon snipped fresh sage or 2 teaspoons dried sage, crushed
- 2 teaspoons ground ancho chile pepper
- ½ teaspoon garlic powder

1. For the remoulade, in a medium bowl combine carrots and sweet potatoes. In a small bowl stir together Paleo Mayo, lemon juice, Dijon-Style Mustard, parsley, and black

pepper. Pour over carrots and sweet potatoes; toss to coat. Cover and chill for 1 to 2 hours.

2. Meanwhile, in a small bowl combine sage, ancho chile, and garlic powder. Rub spice mixture onto lamb chops.

3. For a charcoal or gas grill, place lamb chops on a grill rack directly over medium heat. Cover and grill for 6 to 8 minutes for medium rare (145°F) or 10 to 12 minutes for medium (150°F), turning once halfway through grilling.

4. Serve the lamb chops with the remoulade.

*Note: Use a mandoline with a julienne attachment to cut the sweet potatoes.

LAMB CHOPS WITH SHALLOT, MINT, AND OREGANO RUB

PREP: 20 minutes MARINATE: 1 to 24 hours ROAST: 40 minutes GRILL: 12 minutes MAKES: 4 servings

AS WITH MOST MARINATED MEATS, THE LONGER YOU LEAVE THE HERB RUB ON THE LAMB CHOPS BEFORE COOKING, THE MORE FLAVORFUL THEY WILL BE. THERE IS AN EXCEPTION TO THIS RULE, AND THAT IS WHEN YOU ARE USING A MARINADE THAT CONTAINS HIGHLY ACIDIC INGREDIENTS SUCH AS CITRUS JUICE, VINEGAR, AND WINE. IF YOU LET THE MEAT SIT IN AN ACIDIC MARINADE TOO LONG, IT BEGINS TO BREAK DOWN AND GET MUSHY.

LAMB
- 2 tablespoons finely chopped shallot
- 2 tablespoons finely chopped fresh mint
- 2 tablespoons finely chopped fresh oregano
- 5 teaspoons Mediterranean Seasoning (see recipe)
- 4 teaspoons olive oil
- 2 cloves garlic, minced
- 8 lamb rib chops, cut about 1 inch thick

SALAD
- ¾ pound baby beets, trimmed
- 1 tablespoon olive oil
- ¼ cup fresh lemon juice
- ¼ cup olive oil
- 1 tablespoon finely chopped shallot
- 1 teaspoon Dijon-Style Mustard (see recipe)
- 6 cups mixed greens
- 4 teaspoons snipped chives

1. For the lamb, in a small bowl combine 2 tablespoons shallot, mint, oregano, 4 teaspoons of the Mediterranean seasoning, and 4 teaspoons olive oil. Sprinkle rub over all sides of the lamb chops; rub in with your fingers. Place chops on a plate; cover with plastic wrap and refrigerate for at least 1 hour or up to 24 hours to marinate.

2. For salad, preheat oven to 400°F. Scrub beets well; cut into wedges. Place in a 2-quart baking dish. Drizzle with the 1 tablespoon olive oil. Cover dish with foil. Roast about 40 minutes or until beets are tender. Cool completely. (Beets can be roasted up to 2 days ahead.)

3. In a screw-top jar combine lemon juice, ¼ cup olive oil, 1 tablespoon shallot, Dijon-Style Mustard, and the remaining 1 teaspoon Mediterranean Seasoning. Cover and shake well. In a salad bowl combine beets and greens; toss with some of the vinaigrette.

4. For a charcoal or gas grill, place chops on the greased grill rack directly over medium heat. Cover and grill to desired doneness, turning once halfway through grilling. Allow 12 to 14 minutes for medium rare (145°F) or 15 to 17 minutes for medium (160°F).

5. To serve, place 2 lamb chops and some of the salad on each of four serving plates. Sprinkle with chives. Pass remaining vinaigrette.

GARDEN-STUFFED LAMB BURGERS WITH RED PEPPER COULIS

PREP: 20 minutes STAND: 15 minutes GRILL: 27 minutes MAKES: 4 servings

A COULIS IS NOTHING MORE THAN A SIMPLE, SMOOTH SAUCE MADE FROM PUREED FRUITS OR VEGETABLES. THE BRIGHT AND BEAUTIFUL RED PEPPER SAUCE FOR THESE LAMB BURGERS GETS A DOUBLE DOSE OF SMOKE—FROM GRILLING AND FROM A SHOT OF SMOKED PAPRIKA.

RED PEPPER COULIS
- 1 large red sweet pepper
- 1 tablespoon dry white wine or white wine vinegar
- 1 teaspoon olive oil
- ½ teaspoon smoked paprika

BURGERS
- ¼ cup snipped unsulfured dried tomatoes
- ¼ cup shredded zucchini
- 1 tablespoon snipped fresh basil
- 2 teaspoons olive oil
- ½ teaspoon black pepper
- 1½ pounds ground lamb
- 1 egg white, lightly beaten
- 1 tablespoon Mediterranean Seasoning (see recipe)

1. For the red pepper coulis, place the red pepper on the grill rack directly over medium heat. Cover and grill for 15 to 20 minutes or until charred and very tender, turning the pepper about every 5 minutes to char each side. Remove from the grill and immediately place in a paper bag or foil to completely enclose the pepper. Let stand for 15

minutes or until cool enough to handle. Using a sharp knife, gently pull off skins and discard. Quarter pepper lengthwise and remove stems, seeds, and membranes. In a food processor combine the roasted pepper, wine, olive oil, and smoked paprika. Cover and process or blend until smooth.

2. Meanwhile, for the filling, place dried tomatoes in a small bowl and cover with boiling water. Let stand for 5 minutes; drain. Pat tomatoes and shredded zucchini dry with paper towels. In the small bowl stir together tomatoes, zucchini, basil, olive oil, and ¼ teaspoon of the black pepper; set aside.

3. In a large bowl combine ground lamb, egg white, remaining ¼ teaspoon black pepper, and Mediterranean Seasoning; mix well. Divide meat mixture into eight equal portions and shape each into a ¼-inch-thick patty. Spoon filling onto four of the patties; top with remaining patties and pinch edges to seal in the filling.

4. Place patties on the grill rack directly over medium heat. Cover and grill for 12 to 14 minutes or until done (160°F), turning once halfway through grilling.

5. To serve, top burgers with red pepper coulis.

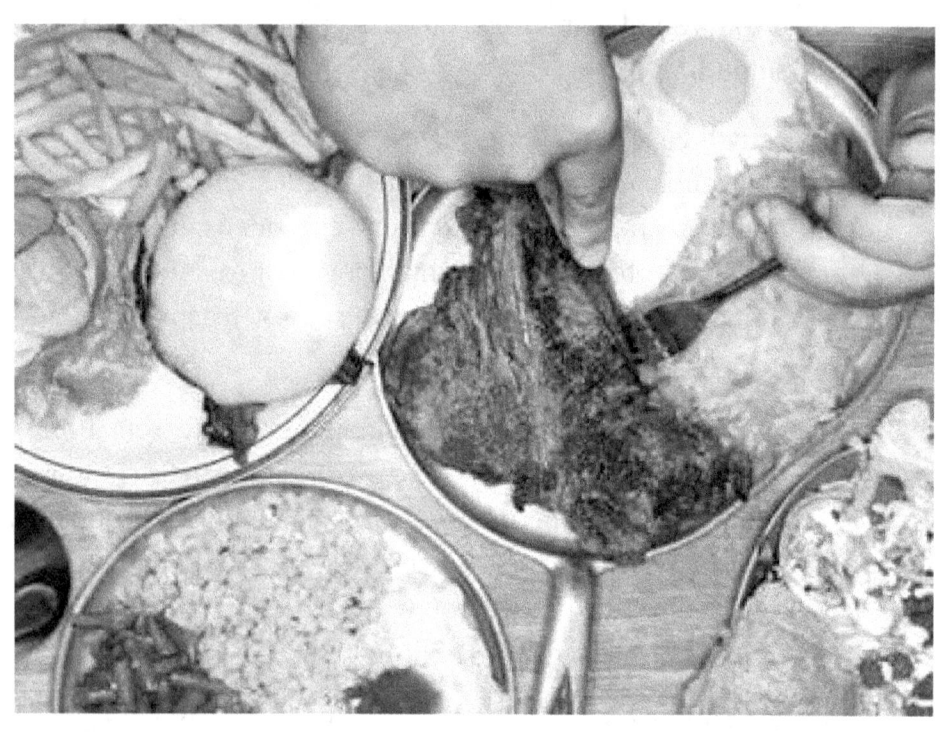

DOUBLE-OREGANO LAMB KABOBS WITH TZATZIKI SAUCE

SOAK: 30 minutes PREP: 20 minutes CHILL: 30 minutes GRILL: 8 minutes MAKES: 4 servings

THESE LAMB KABOBS ARE ESSENTIALLY WHAT IS KNOWN AS KOFTA IN THE MEDITERRANEAN AND MIDDLE EAST—SEASONED GROUND MEAT (USUALLY LAMB OR BEEF) IS SHAPED INTO BALLS OR AROUND A SKEWER AND THEN GRILLED. FRESH AND DRIED OREGANO GIVE THEM GREAT GREEK FLAVOR.

8 10-inch wooden skewers

LAMB KABOBS
1½ pounds lean ground lamb
1 small onion, shredded and squeezed dry
1 tablespoon snipped fresh oregano
2 teaspoon dried oregano, crushed
1 teaspoon black pepper

TZATZIKI SAUCE
1 cup Paleo Mayo (see recipe)
½ of a large cucumber, seeded and shredded and squeezed dry
2 tablespoons fresh lemon juice
1 clove garlic, minced

1. Soak skewers in enough water to cover for 30 minutes.

2. For lamb kabobs, in a large bowl combine ground lamb, onion, fresh and dried oregano, and pepper; mix well. Divide the lamb mixture into eight equal portions. Shape each portion around half of a skewer, creating a 5×1-inch log. Cover and chill for at least 30 minutes.

3. Meanwhile, for Tzatziki Sauce, in a small bowl combine Paleo Mayo, cucumber, lemon juice, and garlic. Cover and chill until serving.

4. For a charcoal or gas grill, place lamb kabobs on grill rack directly over medium heat. Cover and grill about 8 minutes for medium (160°F), turning once halfway through grilling.

5. Serve lamb kabobs with Tzatziki Sauce.

ROAST CHICKEN WITH SAFFRON AND LEMON

PREP: 15 minutes CHILL: 8 hours ROAST: 1 hour 15 minutes STAND: 10 minutes MAKES: 4 servings

SAFFRON IS THE DRIED STAMENS OF A TYPE OF CROCUS FLOWER. IT IS PRICEY, BUT A LITTLE GOES A LONG WAY. IT ADDS ITS EARTHY, DISTINCTIVE FLAVOR AND GORGEOUS YELLOW HUE TO THIS CRISP-SKINNED ROAST CHICKEN.

- 1 4- to 5-pound whole chicken
- 3 tablespoons olive oil
- 6 cloves garlic, crushed and peeled
- 1½ tablespoons finely shredded lemon peel
- 1 tablespoon fresh thyme
- 1½ teaspoons cracked black pepper
- ½ teaspoon saffron threads
- 2 bay leaves
- 1 lemon, quartered

1. Remove neck and giblets from chicken; discard or save for another use. Rinse chicken body cavity; pat dry with paper towels. Snip any excess skin or fat from chicken.

2. In a food processor combine olive oil, garlic, lemon peel, thyme, pepper, and saffron. Process to form a smooth paste.

3. Using fingers, rub paste over the outside surface of the chicken and the inside cavity. Transfer chicken to a large bowl; cover and refrigerate for at least 8 hours or overnight.

4. Preheat oven to 425°F. Place lemon quarters and bay leaves in chicken cavity. Tie legs together with 100%-cotton kitchen string. Tuck wings under chicken. Insert an oven-going meat thermometer into the inside thigh muscle without touching bone. Place chicken on a rack in a large roasting pan.

5. Roast for 15 minutes. Reduce oven temperature to 375°F. Roast about 1 hour more or until juices run clear and thermometer registers 175°F. Tent chicken with foil. Let stand for 10 minutes before carving.

SPATCHCOCKED CHICKEN WITH JICAMA SLAW

PREP: 40 minutes GRILL: 1 hour 5 minutes STAND: 10 minutes MAKES: 4 servings

"SPATCHCOCK" IS AN OLD COOKING TERM THAT'S RECENTLY COME BACK INTO USE TO DESCRIBE THE PROCESS OF SPLITTING A SMALL BIRD—SUCH AS A CHICKEN OR CORNISH HEN—DOWN THE BACK AND THEN OPENING IT AND FLATTENING IT LIKE A BOOK TO HELP IT COOK QUICKLY AND MORE EVENLY. IT'S SIMILAR TO BUTTERFLYING BUT REFERS ONLY TO POULTRY.

CHICKEN
- 1 poblano chile
- 1 tablespoon finely chopped shallot
- 3 cloves garlic, minced
- 1 teaspoon finely shredded lemon peel
- 1 teaspoon finely shredded lime peel
- 1 teaspoon Smoky Seasoning (see recipe)
- ½ teaspoon dried oregano, crushed
- ½ teaspoon ground cumin
- 1 tablespoon olive oil
- 1 3- to 3½-pound whole chicken

SLAW
- ½ of a medium jicama, peeled and cut into julienne strips (about 3 cups)
- ½ cup thinly sliced scallions (4)
- 1 Granny Smith apple, peeled, cored, and cut into julienne strips
- ⅓ cup snipped fresh cilantro
- 3 tablespoons fresh orange juice
- 3 tablespoons olive oil
- 1 teaspoon Lemon-Herb Seasoning (see recipe)

1. For a charcoal grill, arrange medium hot coals on one side of the grill. Place a drip pan under the empty side of the grill. Place poblano on the grill rack directly over medium coals. Cover and grill for 15 minutes or until the poblano is charred on all sides, turning occasionally. Immediately wrap poblano in foil; let stand for 10 minutes. Open foil and cut poblano in half lengthwise; remove stems and seeds (see tip). Using a sharp knife, gently peel off skin and discard. Finely chop the poblano. (For a gas grill, preheat grill; reduce heat to medium. Adjust for indirect cooking. Grill as above over burner that is turned on.)

2. For the rub, in a small bowl combine poblano, shallot, garlic, lemon peel, lime peel, Smoky Seasoning, oregano, and cumin. Stir in oil; mix well to make a paste.

3. To spatchcock the chicken, remove the neck and giblets from chicken (save for another use). Place the chicken, breast side down, on a cutting board. Use kitchen shears to make a lengthwise cut down one side of the backbone, starting from the neck end. Repeat the lengthwise cut to opposite side of the backbone. Remove and discard the backbone. Turn chicken skin side up. Press down between the breasts to break the breast bone so the chicken lies flat.

4. Starting at the neck on one side of the breast, slip your fingers between skin and meat, loosening skin as you work toward the thigh. Free the skin around the thigh. Repeat on the other side. Use your fingers to spread rub over the meat under the skin of the chicken.

5. Place chicken, breast side down, on grill rack over drip pan. Weight with two foil-wrapped bricks or a large cast-iron skillet. Cover and grill for 30 minutes. Turn chicken, bone side down, on rack, weighting again with bricks or skillet. Grill, covered, about 30 minutes more or until chicken is no longer pink (175°F in thigh muscle). Remove chicken from grill; let stand for 10 minutes. (For a gas grill, place chicken on grill rack away from heat. Grill as above.)

6. Meanwhile, for the slaw, in a large bowl combine jicama, scallions, apple, and cilantro. In a small bowl whisk together orange juice, oil, and Lemon-Herb Seasoning. Pour over the jicama mixture and toss to coat. Serve chicken with the slaw.

ROASTED CHICKEN HINDQUARTERS WITH VODKA, CARROT, AND TOMATO SAUCE

PREP: 15 minutes COOK: 15 minutes ROAST: 30 minutes MAKES: 4 servings

VODKA CAN BE MADE FROM SEVERAL DIFFERENT FOODSTUFFS, INCLUDING POTATOES, CORN, RYE, WHEAT, AND BARLEY—EVEN GRAPES. ALTHOUGH THERE ISN'T MUCH VODKA IN THIS SAUCE WHEN YOU DIVIDE IT AMONG FOUR SERVINGS, LOOK FOR VOKDA MADE FROM EITHER POTATOES OR GRAPES TO BE PALEO COMPLIANT.

- 3 tablespoons olive oil
- 4 bone-in chicken hindquarters or meaty chicken pieces, skinned
- 1 28-ounce can no-salt-added plum tomatoes, drained
- ½ cup finely chopped onion
- ½ cup finely chopped carrot
- 3 cloves garlic, minced
- 1 teaspoon Mediterranean Seasoning (see recipe)
- ⅛ teaspoon cayenne pepper
- 1 sprig fresh rosemary
- 2 tablespoons vodka
- 1 tablespoon snipped fresh basil (optional)

1. Preheat oven to 375°F. In an extra-large skillet heat 2 tablespoons of the oil over medium-high heat. Add chicken; cook about 12 minutes or until browned, turning to brown evenly. Place skillet in the preheated oven. Roast, uncovered, for 20 minutes.

2. Meanwhile, for sauce, use kitchen scissors to cut up the tomatoes. In a medium saucepan heat the remaining 1

tablespoon oil over medium heat. Add onion, carrot, and garlic; cook for 3 minutes or until tender, stirring frequently. Stir in snipped tomatoes, Mediterranean Seasoning, cayenne pepper, and rosemary sprig. Bring to boiling over medium-high heat; reduce heat. Simmer, uncovered, for 10 minutes, stirring occasionally. Stir in vodka; cook 1 minute more; remove and discard rosemary sprig.

3. Ladle sauce over chicken in skillet. Return skillet to oven. Roast, covered, about 10 minutes more or until chicken is tender and no longer pink (175°F). If desired, sprinkle with basil.

POULET RÔTI AND RUTABAGA FRITES

PREP: 40 minutes BAKE: 40 minutes MAKES: 4 servings

THE CRISP RUTABAGA FRITES ARE DELICIOUS SERVED WITH THE ROASTED CHICKEN AND ITS ATTENDANT COOKING JUICES—BUT THEY ARE EQUALLY TASTY MADE ON THEIR OWN AND SERVED WITH PALEO KETCHUP (SEE RECIPE) OR SERVED BELGIAN-STYLE WITH PALEO AÏOLI (GARLIC MAYO, SEE RECIPE).

6 tablespoons olive oil

1 tablespoon Mediterranean Seasoning (see recipe)

4 bone-in chicken thighs, skinned (about 1 ¼ pounds total)

4 chicken drumsticks, skinned (about 1 pound total)

1 cup dry white wine

1 cup Chicken Bone Broth (see recipe) or no-salt-added chicken broth

1 small onion, quartered

Olive oil

1½ to 2 pounds rutabagas

2 tablespoons snipped fresh chives

Black pepper

1. Preheat oven to 400°F. In a small bowl combine 1 tablespoon of the olive oil and the Mediterranean Seasoning; rub onto chicken pieces. In an extra-large oven-going skillet heat 2 tablespoons of the oil. Add chicken pieces, meaty sides down. Cook, uncovered, about 5 minutes or until browned. Remove skillet from heat. Turn chicken pieces, browned sides up. Add wine, Chicken Bone Broth, and onion.

2. Place skillet in oven on middle rack. Bake, uncovered, for 10 minutes.

3. Meanwhile, for frites, lightly brush a large baking sheet with olive oil; set aside. Peel rutabagas. Using a sharp knife, cut rutabagas into ½-inch slices. Cut slices lengthwise into ½-inch strips. In a large bowl toss rutabaga strips with the remaining 3 tablespoons oil. Spread rutabaga strips in a single layer on prepared baking sheet; place in oven on top rack. Bake for 15 minutes; turn frites over. Bake chicken for 10 minutes more or until no longer pink (175°F). Remove chicken from oven. Bake frites 5 to 10 minutes or until browned and tender.

4. Remove chicken and onion from skillet, reserving juices. Cover chicken and onion to keep warm. Bring juices to boiling over medium heat; reduce heat. Simmer, uncovered, about 5 minutes more or until juices are slightly reduced.

5. To serve, toss frites with chives and season with pepper. Serve chicken with cooking juices and frites.

TRIPLE-MUSHROOM COQ AU VIN WITH CHIVE MASHED RUTABAGAS

PREP: 15 minutes COOK: 1 hour 15 minutes MAKES: 4 to 6 servings

IF THERE IS ANY GRIT IN THE BOWL AFTER SOAKING THE DRIED MUSHROOMS—AND IT IS LIKELY THAT THERE WILL BE—STRAIN THE LIQUID THROUGH A DOUBLE THICKNESS OF CHEESECLOTH SET IN A FINE-MESH STRAINER.

- 1 ounce dried porcini or morel mushrooms
- 1 cup boiling water
- 2 to 2½ pounds chicken thighs and drumsticks, skinned
- Black pepper
- 2 tablespoons olive oil
- 2 medium leeks, halved lengthwise, rinsed, and thinly sliced
- 2 portobello mushrooms, sliced
- 8 ounces fresh oyster mushrooms, stemmed and sliced, or sliced fresh button mushrooms
- ¼ cup no-salt-added tomato paste
- 1 teaspoon dried marjoram, crushed
- ½ teaspoon dried thyme, crushed
- ½ cup dry red wine
- 6 cups Chicken Bone Broth (see recipe) or no-salt-added chicken broth
- 2 bay leaves
- 2 to 2½ pounds rutabagas, peeled and chopped
- 2 tablespoons snipped fresh chives
- ½ teaspoon black pepper
- Snipped fresh thyme (optional)

1. In a small bowl combine the porcini mushrooms and the boiling water; let stand for 15 minutes. Remove mushrooms, reserving the soaking liquid. Chop the mushrooms. Set the mushrooms and soaking liquid aside.

2. Sprinkle chicken with pepper. In an extra-large skillet with a tight-fitting lid heat 1 tablespoon of the olive oil over medium-high heat. Cook chicken pieces, in two batches, in hot oil about 15 minutes until lightly browned, turning once. Remove chicken from the skillet. Stir in leeks, portobello mushrooms, and oyster mushrooms. Cook for 4 to 5 minutes or just until mushrooms start to brown, stirring occasionally. Stir in tomato paste, marjoram, and thyme; cook and stir for 1 minute. Stir in wine; cook and stir for 1 minute. Stir in 3 cups of the Chicken Bone Broth, bay leaves, ½ cup of the reserved mushroom soaking liquid, and rehydrated chopped mushrooms. Return chicken to skillet. Bring to boiling; reduce heat. Simmer, covered, about 45 minutes or until chicken is tender, turning the chicken once halfway through cooking.

3. Meanwhile, in a large saucepan combine rutabagas and the remaining 3 cups broth. If necessary, add water to just cover rutabagas. Bring to boiling; reduce heat. Simmer, uncovered, for 25 to 30 minutes or until rutabagas are tender, stirring occasionally. Drain rutabagas, reserving liquid. Return rutabagas to the saucepan. Add the remaining 1 tablespoon olive oil, the chives, and the ½ teaspoon pepper. Using a potato masher, mash the rutabaga mixture, adding cooking liquid as needed to make desired consistency.

4. Remove bay leaves from chicken mixture; discard. Serve chicken and sauce over mashed rutabagas. If desired, sprinkle with fresh thyme.

PEACH-BRANDY-GLAZED DRUMSTICKS

PREP: 30 minutes GRILL: 40 minutes MAKES: 4 servings

THESE CHICKEN LEGS ARE PERFECT WITH A CRISPY SLAW AND THE SPICY OVEN-BAKED SWEET POTATO FRIES FROM THE RECIPE FOR TUNISIAN SPICE-RUBBED PORK SHOULDER (SEE RECIPE). THEY'RE SHOWN HERE WITH CRUNCHY CABBAGE SLAW WITH RADISHES, MANGO, AND MINT (SEE RECIPE).

PEACH-BRANDY GLAZE
- 1 tablespoon olive oil
- ½ cup chopped onion
- 2 fresh medium peaches, halved, pitted, and chopped
- 2 tablespoons brandy
- 1 cup BBQ Sauce (see recipe)
- 8 chicken drumsticks (2 to 2½ pounds total), skinned if desired

1. For glaze, in a medium saucepan heat olive oil over medium heat. Add onion; cook about 5 minutes or until tender, stirring occasionally. Add peaches. Cover and cook for 4 to 6 minutes or until peaches are tender, stirring occasionally. Add brandy; cook, uncovered, for 2 minutes, stirring occasionally. Cool slightly. Transfer peach mixture to a blender or food processor. Cover and blend or process until smooth. Add BBQ Sauce. Cover and blend or process until smooth. Return sauce to the saucepan. Cook over medium-low heat just until heated through. Transfer ¾ cup of the sauce to a small bowl for brushing on the chicken. Keep remaining sauce warm for serving with grilled chicken.

2. For a charcoal grill, arrange medium-hot coals around a drip pan. Test for medium heat above drip pan. Place chicken drumsticks on grill rack over drip pan. Cover and grill for 40 to 50 minutes or until chicken is no longer pink (175°F), turning once halfway through grilling and brushing with ¾ cup of the Peach-Brandy Glaze for the last 5 to 10 minutes of grilling. (For a gas grill, preheat grill. Reduce heat to medium. Adjust heat for indirect cooking. Add chicken drumsticks to grill rack that is not over the heat. Cover and grill as directed.)

CHILE-MARINATED CHICKEN WITH MANGO-MELON SALAD

PREP: 40 minutes CHILL/MARINATE: 2 to 4 hours GRILL: 50 minutes MAKES: 6 to 8 servings

AN ANCHO CHILE IS A DRIED POBLANO—A GLOSSY, DEEP-GREEN CHILE WITH AN INTENSELY FRESH FLAVOR. ANCHO CHILES HAVE A SLIGHTLY FRUITY FLAVOR WITH A HINT OF PLUM OR RAISIN AND JUST A TOUCH OF BITTERNESS. NEW MEXICO CHILES CAN BE MODERATELY HOT. THEY'RE THE DEEP-RED CHILES YOU SEE BUNCHED AND HANGING IN RISTRAS—COLORFUL ARRANGEMENTS OF DRYING CHILES—IN PARTS OF THE SOUTHWEST.

CHICKEN
- 2 dried New Mexico chiles
- 2 dried ancho chiles
- 1 cup boiling water
- 3 tablespoons olive oil
- 1 large sweet onion, peeled and cut into thick slices
- 4 roma tomatoes, cored
- 1 tablespoon minced garlic (6 cloves)
- 2 teaspoons ground cumin
- 1 teaspoon dried oregano, crushed
- 16 chicken drumsticks

SALAD
- 2 cups cubed cantaloupe
- 2 cups cubed honeydew
- 2 cups cubed mango
- ¼ cup fresh lime juice
- 1 teaspoon chili powder

½ teaspoon ground cumin

¼ cup snipped fresh cilantro

1. For chicken, remove stems and seeds from dried New Mexico and ancho chiles. Heat a large skillet over medium heat. Toast chiles in the skillet for 1 to 2 minutes or until fragrant and lightly toasted. Place toasted chiles in a small bowl; add the boiling water to the bowl. Let stand at least 10 minutes or until ready to use.

2. Preheat the broiler. Line a baking sheet with foil; brush 1 tablespoon of the olive oil over foil. Place onion slices and tomatoes on pan. Broil about 4 inches from heat for 6 to 8 minutes or until softened and charred. Drain chiles, reserving the water.

3. For marinade, in a blender or food processor combine chiles, onion, tomatoes, garlic, cumin, and oregano. Cover and blend or process until smooth, adding reserved water as needed to puree and reach desired consistency.

4. Place chicken in a large resealable plastic bag set in a shallow dish. Pour marinade over chicken in bag, turning bag to coat evenly. Marinate in refrigerator for 2 to 4 hours, turning bag occasionally.

5. For salad, in an extra-large bowl combine cantaloupe, honeydew, mango, lime juice, the remaining 2 tablespoons olive oil, chili powder, cumin, and cilantro. Toss to coat. Cover and chill for 1 to 4 hours.

6. For a charcoal grill, arrange medium-hot coals around a drip pan. Test for medium heat above the pan. Drain chicken, reserving the marinade. Place chicken on the grill rack over the drip pan. Brush chicken generously with some of

the reserved marinade (discard any extra marinade). Cover and grill for 50 minutes or until chicken is no longer pink (175°F), turning once halfway through grilling. (For a gas grill, preheat grill. Reduce heat to medium. Adjust for indirect cooking. Continue as directed, placing chicken on the burner that is turned off.) Serve chicken drumsticks with salad.

TANDOORI-STYLE CHICKEN LEGS WITH CUCUMBER RAITA

PREP: 20 minutes MARINATE: 2 to 24 hours BROIL: 25 minutes MAKES: 4 servings

THE RAITA IS MADE WITH CASHEW CREAM, LEMON JUICE, MINT, CILANTRO, AND CUCUMBER. IT PROVIDES A COOLING COUNTERPOINT TO THE HOT AND SPICY CHICKEN.

CHICKEN
- 1 onion, cut into thin wedges
- 1 2-inch piece fresh ginger, peeled and quartered
- 4 cloves garlic
- 3 tablespoons olive oil
- 2 tablespoons fresh lemon juice
- 1 teaspoon ground cumin
- 1 teaspoon ground turmeric
- ½ teaspoon ground allspice
- ½ teaspoon ground cinnamon
- ½ teaspoon black pepper
- ¼ teaspoon cayenne pepper
- 8 chicken drumsticks

CUCUMBER RAITA
- 1 cup Cashew Cream (see recipe)
- 1 tablespoon fresh lemon juice
- 1 tablespoon snipped fresh mint
- 1 tablespoon snipped fresh cilantro
- ½ teaspoon ground cumin
- ⅛ teaspoon black pepper
- 1 medium cucumber, peeled, seeded, and diced (1 cup)
- Lemon wedges

1. In a blender or food processor combine onion, ginger, garlic, olive oil, lemon juice, cumin, turmeric, allspice, cinnamon, black pepper, and cayenne pepper. Cover and blend or process until smooth.

2. Using the tip of a paring knife, pierce each drumstick four or five times. Place drumsticks in a large resealable plastic bag set in a large bowl. Add onion mixture; turn to coat. Marinate in the refrigerator for 2 to 24 hours, turning bag occasionally.

3. Preheat broiler. Remove chicken from marinade. Using paper towels, wipe excess marinade from drumsticks. Arrange drumsticks on the rack of an unheated broiler pan or rimmed baking sheet lined with foil. Broil 6 to 8 inches from heat source for 15 minutes. Turn drumsticks over; broil about 10 minutes or until chicken is no longer pink (175°F).

4. For the raita, in a medium bowl combine Cashew Cream, lemon juice, mint, cilantro, cumin, and black pepper. Gently stir in cucumber.

5. Serve chicken with raita and lemon wedges.

CURRIED CHICKEN STEW WITH ROOT VEGETABLES, ASPARAGUS, AND GREEN APPLE-MINT RELISH

PREP: 30 minutes COOK: 35 minutes STAND: 5 minutes MAKES: 4 servings

2 tablespoons refined coconut oil or olive oil
2 pounds bone-in chicken breasts, skinned if desired
1 cup chopped onion
2 tablespoons grated fresh ginger
2 tablespoons minced garlic
2 tablespoons salt-free curry powder
2 tablespoons minced, seeded jalapeño (see tip)
4 cups Chicken Bone Broth (see recipe) or no-salt-added chicken broth
2 medium sweet potatoes (about 1 pound), peeled and chopped
2 medium turnips (about 6 ounces), peeled and chopped
1 cup seeded, diced tomato
8 ounces asparagus, trimmed and cut into 1-inch lengths
1 13.5-ounce can natural coconut milk (such as Nature's Way)
½ cup snipped fresh cilantro
Apple-Mint Relish (see recipe, below)
Lime wedges

1. In a 6-quart Dutch oven heat oil over medium-high heat. Brown chicken in batches in hot oil, turning to brown evenly, about 10 minutes. Transfer chicken to a plate; set aside.

2. Turn heat to medium. Add onion, ginger, garlic, curry powder, and jalapeño to the pot. Cook and stir 5 minutes or until onion is softened. Stir in Chicken Bone Broth, sweet potatoes, turnips, and tomato. Return the chicken pieces to the pot, arranging to submerge chicken in as much liquid as possible. Reduce heat to medium-low.

Cover and simmer 30 minutes or until chicken is no longer pink and vegetables are tender. Stir in asparagus, coconut milk, and cilantro. Remove from heat. Let stand for 5 minutes. Cut chicken from bones, if necessary, to divide evenly among serving bowls. Serve with Apple-Mint Relish and lime wedges.

Apple-Mint Relish: In a food processor chop ½ cup unsweetened coconut flakes until powdery. Add 1 cup fresh cilantro leaves and steams; 1 cup fresh mint leaves; 1 Granny Smith apple, cored and chopped; 2 teaspoons minced, seeded jalapeño (see tip); and 1 tablespoon fresh lime juice. Pulse until finely minced.

GRILLED CHICKEN PAILLARD SALAD WITH RASPBERRIES, BEETS, AND ROASTED ALMONDS

PREP: 30 minutes ROAST: 45 minutes MARINATE: 15 minutes GRILL: 8 minutes MAKES: 4 servings

- ½ cup whole almonds
- 1½ teaspoons olive oil
- 1 medium red beet
- 1 medium golden beet
- 2 6- to 8-ounce boneless, skinless chicken breast halves
- 2 cups fresh or frozen raspberries, thawed
- 3 tablespoons white or red wine vinegar
- 2 tablespoons snipped fresh tarragon
- 1 tablespoon minced shallot
- 1 teaspoon Dijon-Style Mustard (see recipe)
- ¼ cup olive oil
- Black pepper
- 8 cups spring mix lettuces

1. For the almonds, preheat the oven to 400°F. Spread almonds on a small baking sheet and toss with ½ teaspoon olive oil. Bake about 5 minutes or until fragrant and golden. Let cool. (Almonds may be toasted 2 days ahead and stored in an airtight container.)

2. For the beets, place each beet on a small piece of foil and drizzle with each with ½ teaspoon olive oil. Loosely wrap the foil around the beets and place on a baking sheet or in a baking dish. Roast the beets in the 400°F oven for 40 to 50 minutes or until tender when pierced with a knife. Remove from oven and let stand until cool enough to handle. Using a paring knife, remove the skin. Cut beets

into wedges and set aside. (Avoid mixing the beets together to prevent the red beets from staining the golden beets. Beets may be roasted 1 day ahead and chilled. Bring to room temperature before serving.)

3. For the chicken, cut each chicken breast in half horizontally. Place each piece of chicken between two pieces of plastic wrap. Using a meat mallet, gently pound to about ¾ inch thick. Place chicken in a shallow dish and set aside.

4. For vinaigrette, in a large bowl lightly crush ¾ cup of the raspberries with a whisk (reserve remaining raspberries for the salad). Add the vinegar, tarragon, shallot, and Dijon-Style Mustard; whisk to blend. Add the ¼ cup olive oil in a thin stream, whisking to mix well. Pour ½ cup vinaigrette over the chicken; turn chicken to coat (reserve remaining vinaigrette for the salad). Marinate chicken at room temperature for 15 minutes. Remove chicken from the marinade and sprinkle with pepper; discard marinade remaining in dish.

5. For a charcoal or gas grill, place chicken on a grill rack directly over medium heat. Cover and grill for 8 to 10 minutes or until chicken is no longer pink, turning once halfway through grilling. (Chicken can also be cooked in a stovetop grill pan.)

6. In a large bowl combine lettuce, beets, and the remaining 1¼ cups raspberries. Pour reserved vinaigrette over salad; gently toss to coat. Divide salad among four serving plates; top each with a grilled chicken breast piece. Coarsely chop the roasted almonds and sprinkle over all. Serve immediately.

BROCCOLI RABE-STUFFED CHICKEN BREASTS WITH FRESH TOMATO SAUCE AND CAESAR SALAD

PREP: 40 minutes COOK: 25 minutes MAKES: 6 servings

3 tablespoons olive oil

2 teaspoons minced garlic

¼ teaspoon crushed red pepper

1 pound broccoli raab, trimmed and chopped

½ cup unsulfured golden raisins

½ cup water

4 5- to 6-ounce skinless, boneless chicken breast halves

1 cup chopped onion

3 cups chopped tomatoes

¼ cup snipped fresh basil

2 teaspoons red wine vinegar

3 tablespoons fresh lemon juice

2 tablespoons Paleo Mayo (see recipe)

2 teaspoons Dijon-Style Mustard (see recipe)

1 teaspoon minced garlic

½ teaspoon black pepper

¼ cup olive oil

10 cups chopped romaine lettuce

1. In a large skillet heat 1 tablespoon of the olive oil over medium-high heat. Add the garlic and crushed red pepper; cook and stir for 30 seconds or until fragrant. Add the chopped broccoli rabe, raisins, and the ½ cup water. Cover and cook about 8 minutes or until broccoli raab is wilted and tender. Remove lid from pan; let any excess water evaporate. Set aside.

2. For roulades, halve each chicken breast lengthwise; place each piece between two pieces of plastic wrap. Using the flat side of a meat mallet, pound chicken lightly to about ¼ inch thick. For each roulade, place about ¼ cup of the broccoli raab mixture on one of the short ends; roll up, folding in the sides to completely enclose filling. (Roulades may be made up to 1 day ahead and chilled until ready to cook.)

3. In a large skillet heat 1 tablespoon of the olive oil over medium-high heat. Add the roulades, seam sides down. Cook about 8 minutes or until browned on all sides, turning two or three times during cooking. Transfer roulades to a platter.

4. For sauce, in the skillet heat 1 tablespoon of the remaining olive oil over medium heat. Add the onion; cook about 5 minutes or until translucent. Stir in the tomatoes and basil. Place roulades on top of the sauce in skillet. Bring to boiling over medium-high heat; reduce heat. Cover and simmer about 5 minutes or until tomatoes start to break down but still retain their shape and roulades are heated through.

5. For dressing, in a small bowl whisk together the lemon juice, Paleo Mayo, Dijon-Style Mustard, garlic, and black pepper. Drizzle in the ¼ cup olive oil, whisking until emulsified. In a large bowl toss dressing with the chopped romaine. To serve, divide romaine among six serving plates. Slice roulades and arrange on romaine; drizzle with tomato sauce.

GRILLED CHICKEN SHAWARMA WRAPS WITH SPICED VEGETABLES AND PINE NUT DRESSING

PREP: 20 minutes MARINATE: 30 minutes GRILL: 10 minutes MAKES: 8 wraps (4 servings)

1½ pounds skinless, boneless chicken breast halves, cut into 2-inch pieces
5 tablespoons olive oil
2 tablespoons fresh lemon juice
1¾ teaspoons ground cumin
1 teaspoon minced garlic
1 teaspoon paprika
½ teaspoon curry powder
½ teaspoon ground cinnamon
¼ teaspoon cayenne pepper
1 medium zucchini, halved
1 small eggplant cut into ½-inch slices
1 large yellow sweet pepper, halved and seeded
1 medium red onion, quartered
8 cherry tomatoes
8 large butter lettuce leaves
Toasted Pine Nut Dressing (see recipe)
Lemon wedges

1. For marinade, in a small bowl combine 3 tablespoons of the olive oil, lemon juice, 1 teaspoon of the cumin, garlic, ½ teaspoon of the paprika, curry powder, ¼ teaspoon of the cinnamon, and cayenne pepper. Place chicken pieces in a large resealable plastic bag set in a shallow dish. Pour marinade over the chicken. Seal bag; turn bag to coat. Marinate in the refrigerator for 30 minutes, turning bag occasionally.

2. Remove chicken from marinade; discard marinade. Thread chicken on four long skewers.

3. Place zucchini, eggplant, sweet pepper, and onion on a baking sheet. Drizzle with 2 tablespoons of the olive oil. Sprinkle with the remaining ¾ teaspoon cumin, remaining ½ teaspoon paprika, and the remaining ¼ teaspoon cinnamon; lightly rub over vegetables. Thread tomatoes on two skewers.

3. For a charcoal or gas grill, place chicken and tomato kabobs and vegetables on a grill rack over medium heat. Cover and grill until chicken is no longer pink and vegetables are lightly charred and crisp-tender, turning once. Allow 10 to 12 minutes for chicken, 8 to 10 minutes for vegetables, and 4 minutes for tomatoes.

4. Remove chicken from skewers. Chop chicken and cut zucchini, eggplant, and sweet pepper into bite-size pieces. Remove the tomatoes from skewers (do not chop). Arrange chicken and vegetables on a platter. To serve, spoon some of the chicken and vegetables into a lettuce leaf; drizzle with Toasted Pine Nut Dressing. Serve with lemon wedges.

OVEN-BRAISED CHICKEN BREASTS WITH MUSHROOMS, GARLIC-MASHED CAULIFLOWER, AND ROASTED ASPARAGUS

START TO FINISH: 50 minutes MAKES: 4 servings

- 4 10- to 12-ounce bone-in chicken breast halves, skinned
- 3 cups small white button mushrooms
- 1 cup thinly sliced leeks or yellow onion
- 2 cups Chicken Bone Broth (see recipe) or no-salt-added chicken broth
- 1 cup dry white wine
- 1 large bunch fresh thyme
- Black pepper
- White wine vinegar (optional)
- 1 head cauliflower, separated into florets
- 12 cloves garlic, peeled
- 2 tablespoons olive oil
- White or cayenne pepper
- 1 pound asparagus, trimmed
- 2 teaspoons olive oil

1. Preheat oven to 400°F. Arrange chicken breasts in a 3-quart rectangular baking dish; top with mushrooms and leeks. Pour Chicken Bone Broth and wine over the chicken and vegetables. Scatter thyme over all and sprinkle with black pepper. Cover dish with foil.

2. Bake for 35 to 40 minutes or until an instant-read thermometer inserted in chicken registers 170°F. Remove and discard thyme sprigs. If desired, season braising liquid with a splash of vinegar before serving.

2. Meanwhile, in a large saucepan cook cauliflower and garlic in enough boiling water to cover about 10 minutes or until very tender. Drain cauliflower and garlic, reserving 2 tablespoons of the cooking liquid. In a food processor or a large mixing bowl place cauliflower and reserved cooking liquid. Process until smooth* or mash with a potato masher; stir in 2 tablespoons olive oil and season to taste with white pepper. Keep warm until ready to serve.

3. Arrange asparagus in a single layer on a baking sheet. Drizzle with 2 teaspoons olive oil and toss to coat. Sprinkle with black pepper. Roast in a 400°F oven about 8 minutes or until crisp-tender, stirring once.

4. Divide mashed cauliflower among six serving plates. Top with chicken, mushrooms, and leeks. Drizzle with some of the braising liquid; serve with roasted asparagus.

*Note: If using a food processor, be careful not to overprocess or cauliflower will get too thin.

THAI-STYLE CHICKEN SOUP

PREP: 30 minutes FREEZE: 20 minutes COOK: 50 minutes MAKES: 4 to 6 servings

TAMARIND IS A MUSKY, SOUR FRUIT USED IN INDIAN, THAI, AND MEXICAN COOKING. MANY COMMERCIALLY PREPARED TAMARIND PASTES CONTAIN SUGAR—BE SURE YOU PURCHASE ONE THAT DOES NOT. KAFFIR LIME LEAVES CAN BE FOUND FRESH, FROZEN, AND DRIED AT MOST ASIAN MARKETS. IF YOU CAN'T FIND THEM, SUBSTITUTE 1½ TEASPOONS FINELY SHREDDED LIME PEEL FOR THE LEAVES IN THIS RECIPE.

- 2 stalks lemongrass, trimmed
- 2 tablespoons unrefined coconut oil
- ½ cup thinly sliced scallions
- 3 large cloves garlic, thinly sliced
- 8 cups Chicken Bone Broth (see recipe) or no-salt-added chicken broth
- ¼ cup no-sugar-added tamarind paste (such as Tamicon brand)
- 2 tablespoons nori flakes
- 3 fresh Thai chiles, thinly sliced with seeds intact (see tip)
- 3 kaffir lime leaves
- 1 3-inch piece ginger, thinly sliced
- 4 6-ounce skinless, boneless chicken breast halves
- 1 14.5-ounce can no-salt-added fire-roasted diced tomatoes, undrained
- 6 ounces thin asparagus spears, trimmed and thinly sliced diagonally into ½-inch pieces
- ½ cup packed Thai basil leaves (see note)

1. Using the back of a knife with firm pressure, bruise the lemongrass stalks. Finely chop bruised stalks.

2. In a Dutch oven heat coconut oil over medium heat. Add lemongrass and scallions; cook for 8 to 10 minutes,

stirring often. Add garlic; cook and stir for 2 to 3 minutes or until very fragrant.

3. Add Chicken Bone Broth, tamarind paste, nori flakes, chiles, lime leaves, and ginger. Bring to boiling; reduce heat. Cover and simmer for 40 minutes.

4. Meanwhile, freeze chicken for 20 to 30 minutes or until firm. Thinly slice chicken.

5. Strain soup through a fine-mesh sieve into a large saucepan, pressing with the back of a large spoon to extract flavors. Discard solids. Bring soup to boiling. Stir in chicken, undrained tomatoes, asparagus, and basil. Reduce heat; simmer, uncovered, for 2 to 3 minutes or until chicken is cooked through. Serve immediately.

LEMON AND SAGE ROASTED CHICKEN WITH ENDIVE

PREP: 15 minutes ROAST: 55 minutes STAND: 5 minutes MAKES: 4 servings

THE LEMON SLICES AND SAGE LEAF PLACED UNDER THE SKIN OF THE CHICKEN FLAVOR THE MEAT AS IT COOKS—AND MAKE AN EYE-CATCHING DESIGN UNDER THE CRISP, OPAQUE SKIN AFTER IT COMES OUT OF THE OVEN.

- 4 bone-in chicken breast halves (with skin)
- 1 lemon, very thinly sliced
- 4 large sage leaves
- 2 teaspoons olive oil
- 2 teaspoons Mediterranean Seasoning (see recipe)
- ½ teaspoon black pepper
- 2 tablespoons extra virgin olive oil
- 2 shallots, sliced
- 2 cloves garlic, minced
- 4 heads endive, halved lengthwise

1. Preheat oven to 400°F. Using a paring knife, very carefully loosen the skin from each breast half, leaving it attached on one side. Place 2 lemon slices and 1 sage leaf on the meat of each breast. Gently pull skin back into place and press gently to secure it.

2. Arrange chicken in a shallow roasting pan. Brush chicken with 2 teaspoons olive oil; sprinkle with Mediterranean Seasoning and ¼ teaspoon of the pepper. Roast, uncovered, about 55 minutes or until skin is browned and crisp and an instant-read thermometer inserted into

chicken registers 170°F. Let chicken stand for 10 minutes before serving.

3. Meanwhile, in a large skillet heat the 2 tablespoons olive oil over medium heat. Add shallots; cook about 2 minutes or until translucent. Sprinkle endive with the remaining ¼ teaspoon pepper. Add garlic to skillet. Place endive in skillet, cut sides down. Cook about 5 minutes or until browned. Carefully turn endive over; cook for 2 to 3 minutes more or until tender. Serve with chicken.

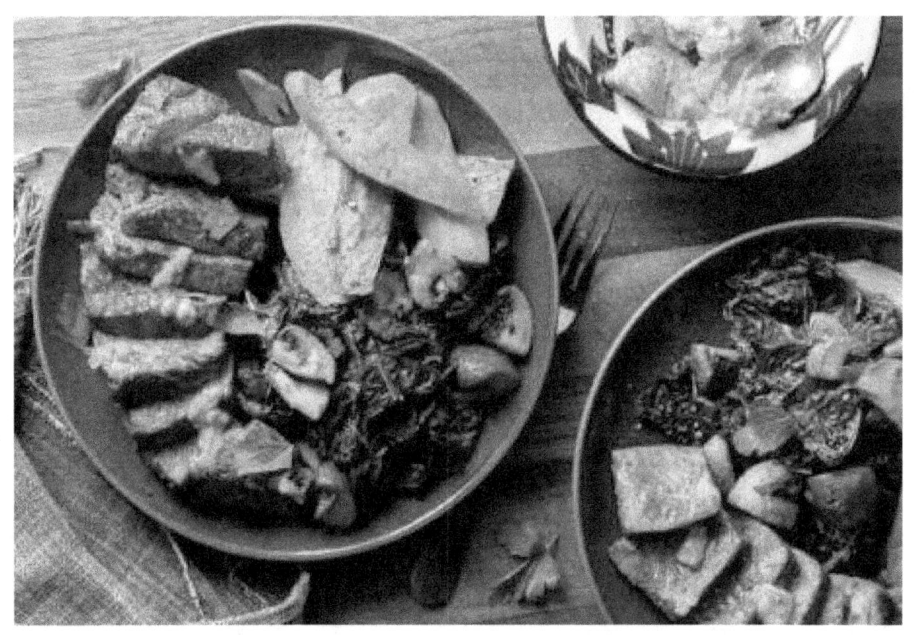

CHICKEN WITH SCALLIONS, WATERCRESS, AND RADISHES

PREP: 20 minutes COOK: 8 minutes BAKE: 30 minutes MAKES: 4 servings

ALTHOUGH IT MIGHT SOUND ODD TO COOK RADISHES, THEY ARE BARELY COOKED HERE—JUST ENOUGH TO MELLOW THEIR PEPPERY BITE AND TENDERIZE THEM A BIT.

3 tablespoons olive oil
4 10- to 12-ounce bone-in chicken breast halves (with skin)
1 tablespoon Lemon-Herb Seasoning (see recipe)
¾ cup sliced scallions
6 radishes, thinly sliced
¼ teaspoon black pepper
½ cup dry white vermouth or dry white wine
⅓ cup Cashew Cream (see recipe)
1 bunch watercress, stems trimmed, roughly chopped
1 tablespoon snipped fresh dill

1. Preheat oven to 350°F. In a large skillet heat olive oil over medium-high heat. Pat chicken dry with a paper towel. Cook chicken, skin sides down, for 4 to 5 minutes or until skin is golden and crisp. Turn chicken over; cook about 4 minutes or until browned. Arrange chicken, skin sides up, in a shallow baking dish. Sprinkle chicken with Lemon-Herb Seasoning. Bake about 30 minutes or until an instant-read thermometer inserted into chicken registers 170°F.

2. Meanwhile, pour all but 1 tablespoon drippings from skillet; return skillet to heat. Add scallions and radishes; cook about 3 minutes or just until scallions wilt. Sprinkle with

pepper. Add vermouth, stirring to scrape up browned bits. Bring to boiling; cook until reduced and slightly thickened. Stir in Cashew Cream; bring to boiling. Remove skillet from heat; add watercress and dill, stirring gently just until watercress wilts. Stir in any chicken juices that have accumulated in the baking dish.

3. Divide scallion mixture among four serving plates; top with chicken.

CHICKEN TIKKA MASALA

PREP: 30 minutes MARINATE: 4 to 6 hours COOK: 15 minutes BROIL: 8 minutes MAKES: 4 servings

THIS WAS INSPIRED BY A VERY POPULAR INDIAN DISH THAT MAY NOT HAVE BEEN CREATED IN INDIA AT ALL, BUT RATHER AT AN INDIAN RESTAURANT IN THE UNITED KINGDOM. TRADITIONAL CHICKEN TIKKA MASALA CALLS FOR CHICKEN TO BE MARINATED IN YOGURT AND THEN COOKED IN A SPICY TOMATO SAUCE SPLASHED WITH CREAM. WITHOUT ANY DAIRY BLUNTING THE FLAVOR OF THE SAUCE, THIS VERSION IS ESPECIALLY CLEAN-TASTING. INSTEAD OF RICE, IT'S SERVED OVER CRISP ZUCCHINI NOODLES.

1½ pounds skinless, boneless chicken thighs or chicken breast halves

¾ cup natural coconut milk (such as Nature's Way)

6 cloves garlic, minced

1 tablespoon grated fresh ginger

1 teaspoon ground coriander

1 teaspoon paprika

1 teaspoon ground cumin

¼ teaspoon ground cardamom

4 tablespoons refined coconut oil

1 cup chopped carrots

1 thinly sliced celery

½ cup chopped onion

2 jalapeño or serrano chiles, seeded (if desired) and finely chopped (see tip)

1 14.5-ounce can no-salt-added fire-roasted diced tomatoes, undrained

1 8-ounce can no-salt-added tomato sauce

1 teaspoon no-salt-added garam masala

3 medium zucchini

½ teaspoon black pepper

Fresh cilantro leaves

1. If using chicken thighs, cut each thigh into three pieces. If using chicken breast halves, cut each breast half into 2-inch pieces, cutting any thick portions in half horizontally to make them thinner. Place chicken in a large resealable plastic bag; set aside. For marinade, in a small bowl combine ½ cup of the coconut milk, the garlic, ginger, coriander, paprika, cumin, and cardamom. Pour marinade over chicken in bag. Seal bag and turn to coat chicken. Place bag in a medium bowl; marinate in the refrigerator for 4 to 6 hours, turning bag occasionally.

2. Preheat broiler. In a large skillet heat 2 tablespoons of the coconut oil over medium heat. Add carrots, celery, and onion; cook for 6 to 8 minutes or until vegetables are tender, stirring occasionally. Add jalapeños; cook and stir for 1 minute more. Add undrained tomatoes and tomato sauce. Bring to boiling; reduce heat. Simmer, uncovered, about 5 minutes or until sauce thickens slightly.

3. Drain chicken, discarding marinade. Arrange chicken pieces in a single layer on the unheated rack of a broiler pan. Broil 5 to 6 inches from the heat for 8 to 10 minutes or until chicken is no longer pink, turning once halfway through broiling. Add cooked chicken pieces and the remaining ¼ cup coconut milk to tomato mixture in skillet. Cook for 1 to 2 minutes or until heated through. Remove from the heat; stir in garam masala.

4. Trim ends off zucchini. Using a julienne cutter, cut zucchini into long thin strips. In an extra-large skillet heat the remaining 2 tablespoons coconut oil over medium-high

heat. Add zucchini strips and black pepper. Cook and stir for 2 to 3 minutes or until zucchini is crisp-tender.

5. To serve, divide zucchini among four serving plates. Top with chicken mixture. Garnish with cilantro leaves.

RAS EL HANOUT CHICKEN THIGHS

PREP: 20 minutes COOK: 40 minutes MAKES: 4 servings

RAS EL HANOUT IS A COMPLEX AND EXOTIC MORROCAN SPICE MIXTURE. THE PHRASE MEANS "HEAD OF THE SHOP" IN ARABIC, WHICH IMPLIES THAT IT IS A UNIQUE BLEND OF THE BEST SPICES THE SPICE SELLER HAS TO OFFER. THERE'S NO SET RECIPE FOR RAS EL HANOUT, BUT IT OFTEN CONTAINS SOME BLEND OF GINGER, ANISE, CINNAMON, NUTMEG, PEPPERCORNS, CLOVES, CARDAMOM, DRIED FLOWERS (SUCH AS LAVENDER AND ROSE), NIGELLA, MACE, GALANGAL, AND TURMERIC.

1 tablespoon ground cumin

2 teaspoons ground ginger

1½ teaspoons black pepper

1½ teaspoons ground cinnamon

1 teaspoon ground coriander

1 teaspoon cayenne pepper

1 teaspoon ground allspice

½ teaspoon ground cloves

¼ teaspoon ground nutmeg

1 teaspoon saffron threads (optional)

4 tablespoons unrefined coconut oil

8 bone-in chicken thighs

1 8-ounce package fresh mushrooms, sliced

1 cup chopped onion

1 cup chopped red, yellow, or green sweet pepper (1 large)

4 roma tomatoes, cored, seeded, and chopped

4 cloves garlic, minced

2 13.5-ounce cans natural coconut milk (such as Nature's Way)

3 to 4 tablespoons fresh lime juice

¼ cup finely snipped fresh cilantro

1. For the ras el hanout, in medium mortar or small bowl combine the cumin, ginger, black pepper, cinnamon, coriander, cayenne pepper, allspice, cloves, nutmeg, and, if desired, saffron. Grind with a pestle or stir with a spoon to mix well. Set aside.

2. In an extra-large skillet heat 2 tablespoons of the coconut oil over medium heat. Sprinkle chicken thighs with 1 tablespoon of the ras el hanout. Add chicken to skillet; cook for 5 to 6 minutes or until browned, turning once halfway through cooking. Remove chicken from skillet; keep warm.

3. In the same skillet heat the remaining 2 tablespoons coconut oil over medium heat. Add mushrooms, onion, sweet pepper, tomatoes, and garlic. Cook and stir about 5 minutes or until vegetables are tender. Stir in coconut milk, lime juice, and 1 tablespoon of the ras el hanout. Return chicken to skillet. Bring to boiling; reduce heat. Simmer, covered, about 30 minutes or until chicken is tender (175°F).

4. Serve chicken, vegetables, and sauce in bowls. Garnish with cilantro.

Note: Store leftover Ras el Hanout in a covered container for up to 1 month.

STAR FRUIT ADOBO CHICKEN THIGHS OVER BRAISED SPINACH

PREP: 40 minutes MARINATE: 4 to 8 hours COOK: 45 minutes MAKES: 4 servings

IF NECESSARY, PAT THE CHICKEN DRY WITH A PAPER TOWEL AFTER IT COMES OUT OF THE MARINADE BEFORE BROWNING IT IN THE SKILLET. ANY LIQUID LEFT ON THE MEAT WILL SPATTER IN THE HOT OIL.

- 8 bone-in chicken thighs (1½ to 2 pounds), skinned
- ¾ cup white or cider vinegar
- ¾ cup fresh orange juice
- ½ cup water
- ¼ cup chopped onion
- ¼ cup snipped fresh cilantro
- 4 cloves garlic, minced
- ½ teaspoon black pepper
- 1 tablespoon olive oil
- 1 star fruit (carambola), sliced
- 1 cup Chicken Bone Broth (see recipe) or no-salt-added chicken broth
- 2 9-ounce packages fresh spinach leaves
- Fresh cilantro leaves (optional)

1. Place chicken in a stainless-steel or enamel Dutch oven; set aside. In a medium bowl combine vinegar, orange juice, the water, onion, ¼ cup snipped cilantro, garlic, and pepper; pour over chicken. Cover and marinate in the refrigerator for 4 to 8 hours.

2. Bring chicken mixture in Dutch oven to boiling over medium-high heat; reduce heat. Cover and simmer for 35 to 40 minutes or until chicken is no longer pink (175°F).

3. In an extra-large skillet heat oil over medium-high heat. With tongs, remove chicken from Dutch oven, shaking gently so cooking liquid drips off; reserve cooking liquid. Brown the chicken on all sides, turning frequently to brown evenly.

4. Meanwhile, for sauce, strain cooking liquid; return to Dutch oven. Bring to boiling. Boil about 4 minutes to reduce and thicken slightly; add star fruit; boil for 1 minute more. Return chicken to the sauce in Dutch oven. Remove from heat; cover to keep warm.

5. Wipe out the skillet. Pour Chicken Bone Broth into skillet. Bring to boiling over medium-high heat; stir in spinach. Reduce heat; simmer for 1 to 2 minutes or until spinach is just wilted, stirring constantly. Using a slotted spoon, transfer spinach to a serving platter. Top with chicken and sauce. If desired, sprinkle with cilantro leaves.

CHICKEN-POBLANO CABBAGE TACOS WITH CHIPOTLE MAYO

PREP: 25 minutes BAKE: 40 minutes MAKES: 4 servings

SERVE THESE MESSY-BUT-TASTY TACOS WITH A FORK TO RETRIEVE ANY OF THE FILLING THAT HAPPENS TO FALL OUT OF THE CABBAGE LEAF WHILE YOU'RE EATING IT.

1 tablespoon olive oil
2 poblano chiles, seeded (if desired) and chopped (see tip)
½ cup chopped onion
3 cloves garlic, minced
1 tablespoon salt-free chili powder
2 teaspoons ground cumin
½ teaspoon black pepper
1 8-ounce can no-salt-added tomato sauce
¾ cup Chicken Bone Broth (see recipe) or no-salt-added chicken broth
1 teaspoon dried Mexican oregano, crushed
1 to 1½ pounds skinless, boneless chicken thighs
10 to 12 medium to large cabbage leaves
Chipotle Paleo Mayo (see recipe)

1. Preheat oven to 350°F. In a large ovenproof skillet heat oil over medium-high heat. Add poblano chiles, onion, and garlic; cook and stir for 2 minutes. Stir in chili powder, cumin, and black pepper; cook and stir for 1 minute more (if necessary, reduce heat to prevent spices from burning).

2. Add tomato sauce, Chicken Bone Broth, and oregano to skillet. Bring to boiling. Carefully place chicken thighs in the tomato mixture. Cover skillet with lid. Bake about 40 minutes or until chicken is tender (175°F), turning chicken once halfway.

3. Remove chicken from skillet; cool slightly. Using two forks, shred chicken into bite-size pieces. Stir shredded chicken into tomato mixture in skillet.

4. To serve, spoon chicken mixture into cabbage leaves; top with Chipotle Paleo Mayo.

CHICKEN STEW WITH BABY CARROTS AND BOK CHOY

PREP: 15 minutes COOK: 24 minutes STAND: 2 minutes MAKES: 4 servings

BABY BOK CHOY IS VERY DELICATE AND CAN GET OVERCOOKED IN A FLASH. TO KEEP IT CRISP AND FRESH-TASTING—NOT WILTED AND SOGGY—BE SURE IT STEAMS IN THE COVERED HOT POT (OFF THE HEAT) FOR NO MORE THAN 2 MINUTES BEFORE YOU SERVE THE STEW.

- 2 tablespoons olive oil
- 1 leek, sliced (white and light green parts)
- 4 cups Chicken Bone Broth (see recipe) or no-salt-added chicken broth
- 1 cup dry white wine
- 1 tablespoon Dijon-Style Mustard (see recipe)
- ½ teaspoon black pepper
- 1 sprig fresh thyme
- 1¼ pounds skinless, boneless chicken thighs, cut into 1-inch pieces
- 8 ounces baby carrots with tops, scrubbed, trimmed, and halved lengthwise, or 2 medium carrots, bias-sliced
- 2 teaspoons finely shredded lemon peel (set aside)
- 1 tablespoon fresh lemon juice
- 2 heads baby bok choy
- ½ teaspoon snipped fresh thyme

1. In a large saucepan heat 1 tablespoon of the olive oil over medium heat. Cook leek in hot oil for 3 to 4 minutes or until wilted. Add Chicken Bone Broth, wine, Dijon-Style Mustard, ¼ teaspoon of the pepper, and thyme sprig. Bring to boiling; reduce heat. Cook for 10 to 12 minutes or until liquid is reduced by about one-third. Discard thyme sprig.

2. Meanwhile, in a Dutch oven heat the remaining 1 tablespoon olive oil over medium-high heat. Sprinkle chicken with the remaining ¼ teaspoon pepper. Cook in hot oil about 3 minutes or until browned, stirring occasionally. Drain fat if necessary. Carefully add the reduced broth mixture to pot, scraping up any brown bits; add carrots. Bring to boiling; reduce heat. Simmer, uncovered, for 8 to 10 minutes or just until carrots are tender. Stir in lemon juice. Cut bok choy in half lengthwise. (If bok choy heads are large, cut into quarters.) Place bok choy on top of chicken in pot. Cover and remove from heat; let stand for 2 minutes.

3. Ladle stew into shallow bowls. Sprinkle with lemon peel and snipped thyme.

CASHEW-ORANGE CHICKEN AND SWEET PEPPER STIR-FRY IN LETTUCE WRAPS

START TO FINISH: 45 minutes MAKES: 4 to 6 servings

YOU WILL FIND TWO TYPES OF COCONUT OIL ON THE SHELVES—REFINED AND EXTRA VIRGIN, OR UNREFINED. AS THE NAME IMPLIES, EXTRA VIRGIN COCONUT OIL IS FROM THE FIRST PRESSING OF THE FRESH, RAW COCONUT. IT IS ALWAYS THE BETTER CHOICE WHEN YOU ARE COOKING OVER MEDIUM OR MEDIUM-HIGH HEAT. REFINED COCONUT OIL HAS A HIGHER SMOKE POINT, SO USE IT ONLY WHEN YOU ARE COOKING OVER HIGH HEAT.

- 1 tablespoon refined coconut oil
- 1½ to 2 pounds skinless, boneless chicken thighs, cut into thin bite-size strips
- 3 red, orange, and/or yellow sweet peppers, stemmed, seeded, and thinly sliced into bite-size strips
- 1 red onion, halved lengthwise and thinly sliced
- 1 teaspoon finely shredded orange peel (set aside)
- ½ cup fresh orange juice
- 1 tablespoon minced fresh ginger
- 3 cloves garlic, minced
- 1 cup unsalted raw cashews, toasted and coarsely chopped (see tip)
- ½ cup sliced green scallions (4)
- 8 to 10 butter or iceberg lettuce leaves

1. In a wok or large skillet heat the coconut oil over high heat. Add chicken; cook and stir for 2 minutes. Add peppers and onion; cook and stir for 2 to 3 minutes or until vegetables just start to soften. Remove the chicken and vegetables from the wok; keep warm.

2. Wipe out wok with paper towel. Add the orange juice to the wok. Cook about 3 minutes or until juice boils and reduces slightly. Add ginger and garlic. Cook and stir for 1 minute. Return the chicken and pepper mixture to the wok. Stir in orange peel, cashews, and scallions. Serve stir-fry on lettuce leaves.

VIETNAMESE COCONUT-LEMONGRASS CHICKEN

START TO FINISH: 30 minutes MAKES: 4 servings

THIS QUICK COCONUT CURRY CAN BE ON THE TABLE IN 30 MINUTES FROM THE TIME YOU START CHOPPING, MAKING IT AN IDEAL MEAL FOR A BUSY WEEKNIGHT.

- 1 tablespoon unrefined coconut oil
- 4 stalks lemongrass (pale parts only)
- 1 3.2-ounce package oyster mushrooms, chopped
- 1 large onion, thinly sliced, rings halved
- 1 fresh jalapeño, seeded and finely chopped (see tip)
- 2 tablespoons minced fresh ginger
- 3 cloves garlic minced
- 1½ pounds skinless, boneless chicken thighs, thinly sliced and cut into bite-size pieces
- ½ cup natural coconut milk (such as Nature's Way)
- ½ cup Chicken Bone Broth (see recipe) or no-salt-added chicken broth
- 1 tablespoon salt-free red curry powder
- ½ teaspoon black pepper
- ½ cup snipped fresh basil leaves
- 2 tablespoons fresh lime juice
- Unsweetened shaved coconut (optional)

1. In an extra-large skillet heat coconut oil over medium heat. Add lemongrass; cook and stir for 1 minute. Add mushrooms, onion, jalapeño, ginger, and garlic; cook and stir for 2 minutes or until onion is just tender. Add chicken; cook about 3 minutes or until chicken is cooked through.

2. In a small bowl combine coconut milk, Chicken Bone Broth, curry powder, and black pepper. Add to chicken mixture in skillet; cook for 1 minute or until the liquid has slightly thickened. Remove from heat; stir in fresh basil and lime juice. If desired, sprinkle servings with coconut.

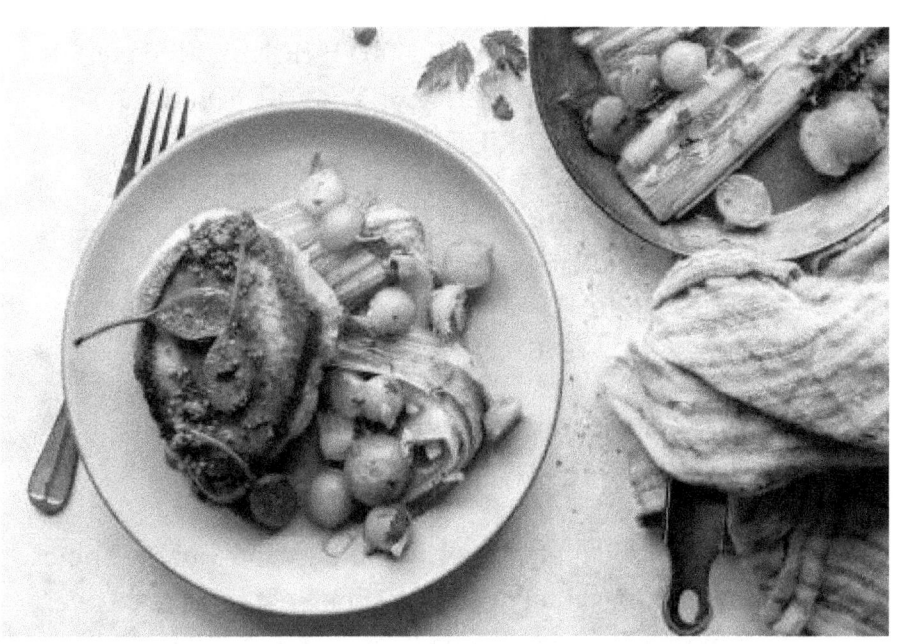

GRILLED CHICKEN AND APPLE ESCAROLE SALAD

PREP: 30 minutes GRILL: 12 minutes MAKES: 4 servings

IF YOU LIKE A SWEETER APPLE, GO WITH HONEYCRISP. IF YOU LIKE A TART APPLE, USE GRANNY SMITH—OR, FOR BALANCE, TRY A MIX OF THE TWO VARIETIES.

- 3 medium Honeycrisp or Granny Smith apples
- 4 teaspoons extra virgin olive oil
- ½ cup finely chopped shallots
- 2 tablespoons snipped fresh parsley
- 1 tablespoon poultry seasoning
- 3 to 4 heads escarole, quartered
- 1 pound ground chicken or turkey breast
- ⅓ cup chopped toasted hazelnuts*
- ⅓ cup Classic French Vinaigrette (see recipe)

1. Halve and core apples. Peel and finely chop 1 of the apples. In a medium skillet heat 1 teaspoon of the olive oil over medium heat. Add chopped apple and shallots; cook until tender. Stir in parsley and poultry seasoning. Set aside to cool.

2. Meanwhile, core the remaining 2 apples and cut into wedges. Brush cut sides of apple wedges and escarole with the remaining olive oil. In a large bowl combine chicken and the cooled apple mixture. Divide into eight portions; shape each portion into a 2-inch-diameter patty.

3. For a charcoal or gas grill, place chicken patties and apple wedges on a grill rack directly over medium heat. Cover and grill for 10 minutes, turning once halfway through

grilling. Add escarole, cut sides down. Cover and grill for 2 to 4 minutes or until escarole is lightly charred, apples are tender, and chicken patties are done (165°F).

4. Coarsely chop escarole. Divide escarole among four serving plates. Top with chicken patties, apple slices, and hazelnuts. Drizzle with Classic French Vinaigrette.

*Tip: To toast hazelnuts, preheat oven to 350°F. Spread nuts in a single layer in a shallow baking pan. Bake for 8 to 10 minutes or until lightly toasted, stirring once to toast evenly. Cool nuts slightly. Place the warm nuts on a clean kitchen towel; rub with the towel to remove the loose skins.

TUSCAN CHICKEN SOUP WITH KALE RIBBONS

PREP: 15 minutes COOK: 20 minutes MAKES: 4 to 6 servings

A SPOONFUL OF PESTO—YOUR CHOICE OF EITHER BASIL OR ARUGULA—ADDS GREAT TASTE TO THIS SAVORY SOUP SEASONED WITH SALT-FREE POULTRY SEASONING. TO KEEP THE KALE RIBBONS BRIGHT GREEN AND AS FULL OF NUTRIENTS AS POSSIBLE, COOK THEM ONLY UNTIL THEY WILT.

- 1 pound ground chicken
- 2 tablespoons no-salt-added poultry seasoning
- 1 teaspoon finely shredded lemon peel
- 1 tablespoon olive oil
- 1 cup chopped onion
- ½ cup chopped carrots
- 1 cup chopped celery
- 4 cloves garlic, sliced
- 4 cups Chicken Bone Broth (see recipe) or no-salt-added chicken broth
- 1 14.5-ounce can no-salt-added fire-roasted tomatoes, undrained
- 1 bunch Lacinato (Tuscan) kale, stems removed, cut into ribbons
- 2 tablespoons fresh lemon juice
- 1 teaspoon snipped fresh thyme
- Basil or Arugula Pesto (see recipes)

1. In a medium bowl combine ground chicken, poultry seasoning, and lemon peel. Mix well.

2. In a Dutch oven heat olive oil over medium heat. Add chicken mixture, onion, carrots, and celery; cook for 5 to 8 minutes or until chicken is no longer pink, stirring with a wooden spoon to break up meat and adding garlic slices the last 1 minute of cooking. Add Chicken Bone Broth and

tomatoes. Bring to boiling; reduce heat. Cover and simmer for 15 minutes. Stir in kale, lemon juice, and thyme. Simmer, uncovered, about 5 minutes or until kale is just wilted.

3. To serve, ladle soup into serving bowls and top with Basil or Arugula Pesto.

CHICKEN LARB

PREP: 15 minutes COOK: 8 minutes COOL: 20 minutes MAKES: 4 servings

THIS VERSION OF THE POPULAR THAI DISH OF HIGHLY SEASONED GROUND CHICKEN AND VEGETABLES SERVED IN LETTUCE LEAVES IS INCREDIBLY LIGHT AND FLAVORFUL—WITHOUT THE ADDITION OF THE SUGAR, SALT, AND FISH SAUCE (WHICH IS VERY HIGH IN SODIUM) THAT ARE TRADITIONALLY PART OF THE INGREDIENTS LIST. WITH GARLIC, THAI CHILES, LEMONGRASS, LIME PEEL, LIME JUICE, MINT, AND CILANTRO, YOU WON'T MISS THEM.

- 1 tablespoon refined coconut oil
- 2 pounds ground chicken (95% lean or ground breast)
- 8 ounces button mushrooms, finely chopped
- 1 cup finely chopped red onion
- 1 to 2 Thai chiles, seeded and finely chopped (see tip)
- 2 tablespoons minced garlic
- 2 tablespoons finely chopped lemongrass*
- ¼ teaspoon ground cloves
- ¼ teaspoon black pepper
- 1 tablespoon finely shredded lime peel
- ½ cup fresh lime juice
- ⅓ cup tightly packed fresh mint leaves, chopped
- ⅓ cup tightly packed fresh cilantro, chopped
- 1 head iceberg lettuce, separated into leaves

1. In an extra-large skillet heat coconut oil over medium-high heat. Add ground chicken, mushrooms, onion, chile(s), garlic, lemongrass, cloves, and black pepper. Cook for 8 to 10 minutes or until chicken is cooked through, stirring with a wooden spoon to break up meat as it cooks. Drain if necessary. Transfer chicken mixture to an extra-large

bowl. Let cool about 20 minutes or until slightly warmer than room temperature, stirring occasionally.

2. Stir lime peel, lime juice, mint, and cilantro into chicken mixture. Serve in lettuce leaves.

*Tip: To prepare the lemongrass, you'll need a sharp knife. Cut the woody stem off of the bottom of the stalk and the tough green blades at the top of the plant. Remove the two tough outer layers. You should have a piece of lemongrass that is about 6 inches long and pale yellow-white. Cut the stalk in half horizontally, then cut each half in half again. Slice each quarter of the stalk very thinly.

CHICKEN BURGERS WITH SZECHWAN CASHEW SAUCE

PREP: 30 minutes COOK: 5 minutes GRILL: 14 minutes MAKES: 4 servings

THE CHILI OIL MADE BY WARMING OLIVE OIL WITH CRUSHED RED PEPPER CAN BE USED IN OTHER WAYS AS WELL. USE IT TO SAUTÉ FRESH VEGETABLES—OR TOSS THEM WITH SOME CHILI OIL BEFORE ROASTING.

- 2 tablespoons olive oil
- ¼ teaspoon crushed red pepper
- 2 cups raw cashew pieces, toasted (see tip)
- ¼ cup olive oil
- ½ cup shredded zucchini
- ¼ cup finely chopped chives
- 2 cloves garlic, minced
- 2 teaspoons finely shredded lemon peel
- 2 teaspoons grated fresh ginger
- 1 pound ground chicken or turkey breast

SZECHWAN CASHEW SAUCE

- 1 tablespoon olive oil
- 2 tablespoons finely chopped scallions
- 1 tablespoon grated fresh ginger
- 1 teaspoon Chinese five-spice powder
- 1 teaspoon fresh lime juice
- 4 green leaf or butter lettuce leaves

1. For the chili oil, in a small saucepan combine the olive oil and the crushed red pepper. Warm over low heat for 5 minutes. Remove from heat; let cool.

2. For cashew butter, place cashews and 1 tablespoon of the olive oil in a blender. Cover and blend until creamy,

stopping to scrape down the sides as needed and adding additional olive oil, 1 tablespoon at a time, until the entire ¼ cup has been used and the butter is very soft; set aside.

3. In a large bowl combine the zucchini, chives, garlic, lemon peel, and the 2 teaspoons ginger. Add ground chicken; mix well. Shape chicken mixture into four ½-inch-thick patties.

4. For a charcoal or gas grill, place patties on the greased rack directly over medium heat. Cover and grill for 14 to 16 minutes or until done (165°F), turning once halfway through grilling.

5. Meanwhile, for the sauce, in a small skillet heat the olive oil over medium heat. Add the scallions and the 1 tablespoon ginger; cook over medium-low heat for 2 minutes or until scallions soften. Add ½ cup of the cashew butter (refrigerate remaining cashew butter for up to 1 week), chili oil, lime juice, and five-spice powder. Cook for 2 more minutes. Remove from heat.

6. Serve patties on the lettuce leaves. Drizzle with sauce.

TURKISH CHICKEN WRAPS

PREP: 25 minutes STAND: 15 minutes COOK: 8 minutes MAKES: 4 to 6 servings

"BAHARAT" SIMPLY MEANS "SPICE" IN ARABIC. AN ALL-PURPOSE SEASONING IN MIDDLE EASTERN CUISINE, IT IS OFTEN USED AS A RUB ON FISH, POULTRY, AND MEATS OR MIXED WITH OLIVE OIL AND USED AS A VEGETABLE MARINADE. THE COMBINATION OF WARM, SWEET SPICES SUCH AS CINNAMON, CUMIN, CORIANDER, CLOVES, AND PAPRIKA MAKES IT PARTICULARLY AROMATIC. THE ADDITION OF DRIED MINT IS A TURKISH TOUCH.

⅓ cup snipped unsulfured dried apricots
⅓ cup snipped dried figs
1 tablespoon unrefined coconut oil
1½ pounds ground chicken breast
3 cups sliced leeks (white and light green parts only) (3)
⅔ of a medium green and/or red sweet peppers, thinly sliced
2 tablespoons Baharat Seasoning (see recipe, below)
2 cloves garlic, minced
1 cup chopped, seeded tomatoes (2 medium)
1 cup chopped, seeded cucumber (½ of a medium)
½ cup chopped shelled unsalted pistachios, toasted (see tip)
¼ cup snipped fresh mint
¼ cup snipped fresh parsley
8 to 12 large butterhead or Bibb lettuce leaves

1. Place apricots and figs in a small bowl. Add ⅔ cup boiling water; let stand for 15 minutes. Drain, reserving ½ cup of the liquid.

2. Meanwhile, in an extra-large skillet heat coconut oil over medium heat. Add ground chicken; cook for 3 minutes,

stirring with a wooden spoon to break up meat as it cooks. Add leeks, sweet pepper, Baharat Seasoning, and garlic; cook and stir about 3 minutes or until chicken is done and pepper is just tender. Add apricots, figs, reserved liquid, tomatoes, and cucumber. Cook and stir about 2 minutes or until tomatoes and cucumber just start to break down. Stir in pistachios, mint, and parsley.

3. Serve chicken and vegetables in lettuce leaves.

Baharat Seasoning: In a small bowl combine 2 tablespoons sweet paprika; 1 tablespoon black pepper; 2 teaspoons dried mint, finely crushed; 2 teaspoons ground cumin; 2 teaspoons ground coriander; 2 teaspoons ground cinnamon; 2 teaspoons ground cloves; 1 teaspoon ground nutmeg; and 1 teaspoon ground cardamom. Store in a tightly sealed container at room temperature. Makes about ½ cup.

SPANISH CORNISH HENS

PREP: 10 minutes BAKE: 30 minutes BROIL: 6 minutes MAKES: 2 to 3 servings

THIS RECIPE COULD NOT BE EASIER—AND THE RESULTS ARE ABSOLUTELY AMAZING. COPIOUS AMOUNTS OF SMOKED PAPRIKA, GARLIC, AND LEMON GIVE THESE DIMINUTIVE BIRDS BIG FLAVOR.

- 2 1½-pound Cornish hens, thawed if frozen
- 1 tablespoon olive oil
- 6 cloves garlic, chopped
- 2 to 3 tablespoons smoked sweet paprika
- ¼ to ½ teaspoon cayenne pepper (optional)
- 2 lemons, quartered
- 2 tablespoons snipped fresh parsley (optional)

1. Preheat oven to 375°F. To quarter the game hens, use kitchen shears or a sharp knife to cut along both sides of the narrow backbone. Butterfly the bird open and cut the hen in half through the breastbone. Remove the hindquarters by cutting through the skin and meat that separates the thighs from the breast. Keep the wing and breast intact. Rub olive oil over Cornish hen pieces. Sprinkle with chopped garlic.

2. Place the hen pieces, skin sides up, in an extra-large oven-going skillet. Sprinkle with smoked paprika and cayenne. Squeeze the lemon quarters over the hens; add lemon quarters to the skillet. Turn hen pieces skin sides down in the pan. Cover and bake for 30 minutes. Remove skillet from oven.

3. Preheat broiler. Using tongs, turn the pieces. Adjust oven rack. Broil 4 to 5 inches from the heat for 6 to 8 minutes until skin is browned and hens are done (175°F). Drizzle with pan juices. If desired, sprinkle with parsley.

PISTACHIO-ROASTED CORNISH HENS WITH ARUGULA, APRICOT, AND FENNEL SALAD

PREP: 30 minutes CHILL: 2 to 12 hours ROAST: 50 minutes STAND: 10 minutes MAKES: 8 servings

A PISTACHIO PESTO MADE WITH PARSLEY, THYME, GARLIC, ORANGE PEEL, ORANGE JUICE, AND OLIVE OIL IS TUCKED UNDER THE SKIN OF EACH BIRD BEFORE MARINATING.

- 4 20- to 24-ounce Cornish game hens
- 3 cups raw pistachio nuts
- 2 tablespoons snipped fresh Italian (flat-leaf) parsley
- 1 tablespoon snipped thyme
- 1 large clove garlic, minced
- 2 teaspoons finely shredded orange peel
- 2 tablespoons fresh orange juice
- ¾ cup olive oil
- 2 large onions, thinly sliced
- ½ cup fresh orange juice
- 2 tablespoons fresh lemon juice
- ¼ teaspoon freshly ground black pepper
- ¼ teaspoon dry mustard
- 2 5-ounce packages arugula
- 1 large bulb fennel, thinly shaved
- 2 tablespoons snipped fennel fronds
- 4 apricots, pitted and cut into thin wedges

1. Rinse inside cavities of Cornish game hens. Tie legs together with 100%-cotton kitchen string. Tuck wings under bodies; set aside.

2. In a food processor or blender combine pistachios, parsley, thyme, garlic, orange peel, and orange juice. Process until coarse paste forms. With processor running, add ¼ cup of the olive oil in a slow, steady stream.

3. Using fingers, loosen skin on the breast side of a hen to make a pocket. Spread one-fourth of the pistachio mixture evenly under the skin. Repeat with remaining hens and pistachio mixture. Spread sliced onions over bottom of roasting pan; place hens, breast sides up, on top of onions. Cover and refrigerate for 2 to 12 hours.

4. Preheat oven to 425°F. Roast hens for 30 to 35 minutes or until an instant-read thermometer inserted in an inside thigh muscle registers 175°F.

5. Meanwhile, for dressing, in a small bowl combine orange juice, lemon juice, pepper, and mustard. Mix well. Add the remaining ½ cup olive oil in a slow steady stream, whisking constantly.

6. For salad, in a large bowl combine arugula, fennel, fennel fronds, and apricots. Drizzle lightly with dressing; toss well. Reserve additional dressing for another purpose.

7. Remove hens from oven; tent loosely with foil and let stand 10 minutes. To serve, divide the salad evenly among eight serving plates. Cut hens in half lengthwise; place hen halves on salads. Serve immediately.

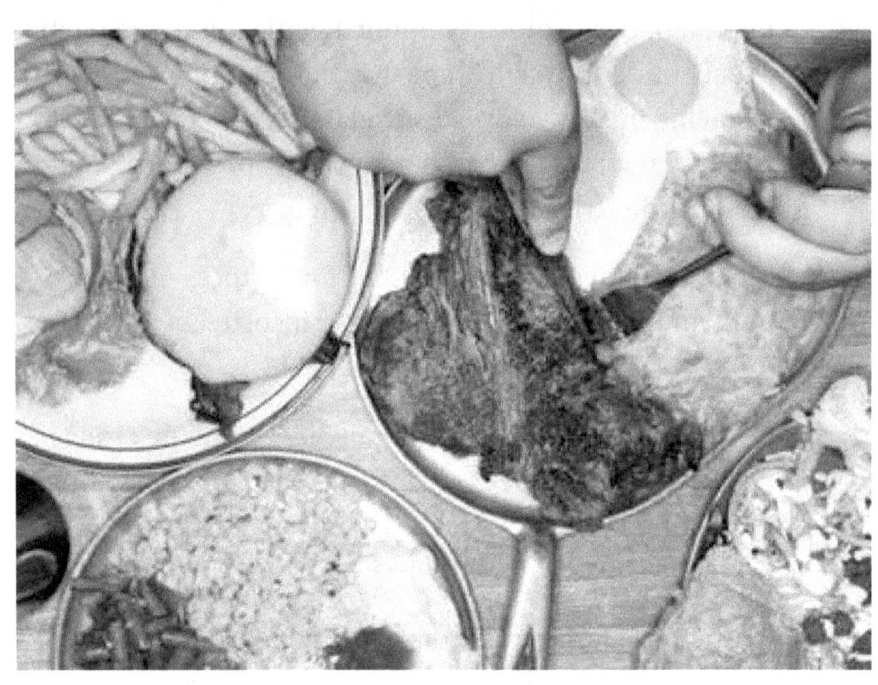

DUCK BREAST WITH POMEGRANATE AND JICAMA SALAD

PREP: 15 minutes COOK: 15 minutes MAKES: 4 servings

CUTTING A DIAMOND PATTERN INTO THE FAT OF THE DUCK BREASTS ALLOWS THE FAT TO RENDER OUT AS THE GARAM MASALA-SEASONED BREASTS COOK. THE DRIPPINGS ARE COMBINED WITH JICAMA, POMEGRANATE SEEDS, ORANGE JUICE, AND BEEF BROTH AND TOSSED WITH PEPPERY GREENS TO WILT THEM JUST SLIGHTLY.

4 boneless Muscovy duck breasts (about 1½ to 2 pounds total)
1 tablespoon garam masala
1 tablespoon unrefined coconut oil
2 cups diced, peeled jicama
½ cup pomegranate seeds
¼ cup fresh orange juice
¼ cup Beef Bone Broth (see recipe) or no-salt-added beef broth
3 cups watercress, stems removed
3 cups torn frisée and/or thinly sliced Belgian endive

1. With a sharp knife, make shallow cuts in diamond patterns into the fat of duck breasts at 1-inch intervals. Sprinkle both sides of the breast halves with the garam masala. Heat an extra-large skillet over medium heat. Melt the coconut oil in the hot skillet. Place breast halves, skin sides down, in the skillet. Cook for 8 minutes with the skin sides down, being careful not to brown too quickly (reduce heat if necessary). Turn duck breasts over; cook for 5 to 6 minutes more or until an instant-read thermometer inserted into breast halves registers 145°F

for medium. Remove breast halves, reserving drippings in a skillet; cover with foil to keep warm.

2. For dressing, add jicama to drippings in skillet; cook and stir for 2 minutes over medium heat. Add pomegranate seeds, orange juice, and Beef Bone Broth to skillet. Bring to boiling; immediately remove from heat.

3. For salad, in a large bowl combine watercress and frisée. Pour hot dressing over greens; toss to coat.

4. Divide salad among four dinner plates. Thinly slice the duck breasts and arrange on salads.

GRILLED STRIP STEAKS WITH GRATED ROOT VEGETABLE HASH

PREP: 20 minutes STAND: 20 minutes GRILL: 10 minutes STAND: 5 minutes MAKES: 4 servings

STRIP STEAKS HAVE A VERY TENDER TEXTURE, AND THE SMALL STRIP OF FAT ON ONE SIDE OF THE STEAK GETS CRISP AND SMOKY ON THE GRILL. MY THINKING ABOUT ANIMAL FAT HAS CHANGED SINCE MY FIRST BOOK. IF YOU ARE FAITHFUL TO THE BASIC PRINCIPLES OF THE PALEO DIET® AND KEEP SATURATED FATS WITHIN 10 TO 15 PERCENT OF YOUR DAILY CALORIES, IT WILL NOT INCREASE YOUR RISK OF HEART DISEASE—AND IN FACT, THE OPPOSITE MAY BE TRUE. NEW INFORMATION SUGGESTS THAT ELEVATIONS IN LDL CHOLESTEROL MAY ACTUALLY REDUCE SYSTEMIC INFLAMMATION, WHICH IS A RISK FACTOR FOR HEART DISEASE.

- 3 tablespoons extra virgin olive oil
- 2 tablespoons grated fresh horseradish
- 1 teaspoon finely shredded orange peel
- ½ teaspoon ground cumin
- ½ teaspoon black pepper
- 4 strip steaks (also called top loin), cut about 1 inch thick
- 2 medium parsnips, peeled
- 1 large sweet potato, peeled
- 1 medium turnip, peeled
- 1 or 2 shallots, finely chopped
- 2 cloves garlic, minced
- 1 tablespoon snipped fresh thyme

1. In a small bowl stir together 1 tablespoon of the oil, horseradish, orange peel, cumin, and ¼ teaspoon of the

pepper. Spread the mixture over steaks; cover and let stand at room temperature for 15 minutes.

2. Meanwhile for hash, using a box grater or a food processor fitted with the shredding blade, shred the parsnips, sweet potato, and turnip. Place shredded vegetables in a large bowl; add shallot(s). In a small bowl combine the remaining 2 tablespoons oil, the remaining ¼ teaspoon pepper, garlic, and thyme. Drizzle over vegetables; toss to mix thoroughly. Fold a 36×18-inch piece of heavy foil in half to make a double thickness of foil that measures 18×18 inches. Place vegetable mixture in the center of the foil; bring up opposite edges of foil and seal with a double fold. Fold remaining edges to completely enclose the vegetables, leaving space for steam to build.

3. For a charcoal or gas grill, place steaks and foil packet on the grill rack directly over medium heat. Cover and grill steaks for 10 to 12 minutes for medium rare (145°F) or 12 to 15 minutes for medium (160°F), turning once halfway through grilling. Grill packet for 10 to 15 minutes or until vegetables are tender. Let steaks stand for 5 minutes while vegetables finish cooking. Divide vegetable hash among four serving plates; top with steaks.

ASIAN BEEF AND VEGETABLE STIR-FRY

PREP: 30 minutes COOK: 15 minutes MAKES: 4 servings

FIVE-SPICE POWDER IS A SALT-FREE SPICE BLEND USED WIDELY IN CHINESE COOKING. IT CONSISTS OF EQUAL PARTS GROUND CINNAMON, CLOVES, FENNEL SEEDS, STAR ANISE, AND SZECHWAN PEPPERCORNS.

- 1½ pounds boneless beef top sirloin steak or boneless beef round steak, cut 1 inch thick
- 1½ teaspoons five-spice powder
- 3 tablespoons refined coconut oil
- 1 small red onion, cut into thin wedges
- 1 small bunch asparagus (about 12 ounces), trimmed and cut into 3-inch pieces
- 1½ cups julienne-cut orange and/or yellow carrots
- 4 cloves garlic, minced
- 1 teaspoon finely shredded orange peel
- ¼ cup fresh orange juice
- ¼ cup Beef Bone Broth (see recipe) or no-salt-added beef broth
- ¼ cup white wine vinegar
- ¼ to ½ teaspoon crushed red pepper
- 8 cups coarsely shredded napa cabbage
- ½ cup unsalted slivered almonds or unsalted coarsely chopped cashews, toasted (see tip, page 57)

1. If desired, partially freeze beef for easier slicing (about 20 minutes). Cut beef into very thin slices. In a large bowl toss together beef and five-spice powder. In a large wok or extra-large skillet heat 1 tablespoon of the coconut oil over medium-high heat. Add half the beef; cook and stir for 3 to 5 minutes or until browned. Transfer beef to a bowl. Repeat with the remaining beef and another 1

tablespoon oil. Transfer beef to the bowl with the other cooked beef.

2. In the same wok add the remaining 1 tablespoon oil. Add onion; cook and stir for 3 minutes. Add asparagus and carrots; cook and stir for 2 to 3 minutes or until vegetables are crisp-tender. Add garlic; cook and stir for 1 minute more.

3. For sauce, in a small bowl combine orange peel, orange juice, Beef Bone Broth, vinegar, and crushed red pepper. Add sauce and all the beef with juices in bowl to vegetables in wok. Cook and stir for 1 to 2 minutes or until heated through. Using a slotted spoon, transfer beef vegetables to a large bowl. Cover to keep warm.

4. Cook the sauce, uncovered, over medium heat for 2 minutes. Add cabbage; cook and stir for 1 to 2 minutes or until cabbage is just wilted. Divide cabbage and any cooking juices among four serving plates. Top evenly with beef mixture. Sprinkle with nuts.

CEDAR-PLANKED FILETS WITH ASIAN SLATHER AND SLAW

SOAK: 1 hour PREP: 40 minutes GRILL: 13 minutes STAND: 10 minutes MAKES: 4 servings.

NAPA CABBAGE IS SOMETIMES CALLED CHINESE CABBAGE. IT HAS BEAUTIFUL, CRINKLY CREAM-COLOR LEAVES WITH BRIGHT YELLOW-GREEN TIPS. IT HAS A DELICATE, MILD FLAVOR AND TEXTURE—QUITE DIFFERENT THAN THE WAXY LEAVES OF ROUND-HEADED CABBAGE—AND NOT SURPRISINGLY, IS A NATURAL IN ASIAN-STYLE DISHES.

1 large cedar plank
¼ ounce dried shiitake mushrooms
¼ cup walnut oil
2 teaspoons minced fresh ginger
2 teaspoons crushed red pepper
1 teaspoon crushed Szechwan peppercorns
¼ teaspoon five-spice powder
4 cloves garlic, minced
4 4- to 5-ounce beef tenderloin steaks, cut ¾ to 1 inch thick
Asian Slaw (see recipe, below)

1. Place grill plank in water; weight down and soak for at least 1 hour.

2. Meanwhile, for Asian slather, in a small bowl pour boiling water over dried shiitake mushrooms; let stand for 20 minutes to rehydrate. Drain mushrooms and place in a food processor. Add walnut oil, ginger, crushed red pepper, Szechuan peppercorns, five-spice powder, and garlic. Cover and process until mushrooms are minced and ingredients are combined; set aside.

3. Drain grill plank. For a charcoal grill, arrange medium-hot coals around perimeter of grill. Place plank on grill rack directly over coals. Cover and grill for 3 to 5 minutes or until plank begins to crackle and smoke. Place steaks on grill rack directly over coals; grill for 3 to 4 minutes or until seared. Transfer steaks to the plank, seared sides up. Place plank in center of grill. Divide Asian Slather among steaks. Cover and grill for 10 to 12 minutes or until an instant-read thermometer inserted horizontally into the steaks reads 130°F. (For a gas grill, preheat grill. Reduce heat to medium. Place drained plank on grill rack; cover and grill for 3 to 5 minutes or until plank begins to crackle and smoke. Place steaks on grill rack for 3 to 4 minutes or until seared. Transfer steaks to the plank, seared sides up. Adjust grill for indirect cooking; place plank with steaks over the burner that is turned off. Divide slather among steaks. Cover and grill for 10 to 12 minutes or until an instant-read thermometer inserted horizontally into the steaks reads 130°F.)

4. Remove steaks from the grill. Cover steaks loosely with foil; let stand for 10 minutes. Cut steaks into ¼-inch-thick slices. Serve steak over Asian Slaw.

Asian Slaw: In a large bowl combine 1 medium head napa cabbage, thinly sliced; 1 cup finely shredded red cabbage; 2 carrots, peeled and cut into julienne strips; 1 red or yellow sweet pepper, seeded and very thinly sliced; 4 scallions, thinly bias-sliced; 1 to 2 serrano chiles, seeded and minced (see tip); 2 tablespoons chopped cilantro; and 2 tablespoons chopped mint. For dressing, in a food processor or blender combine 3 tablespoons fresh lime juice, 1 tablespoon grated fresh ginger, 1 cloves minced garlic, and ⅛ teaspoon five-spice powder. Cover and process until smooth. With the processor running, gradually add ½ cup walnut oil and process until smooth. Add 1 scallion, thinly bias-sliced, to the dressing. Drizzle over slaw and toss to coat.

PAN-SEARED TRI-TIP STEAKS WITH CAULIFLOWER PEPERONATA

PREP: 25 minutes COOK: 25 minutes MAKES: 2 servings

PEPERONATA IS TRADITIONALLY A SLOW-ROASTED RAGU OF SWEET PEPPERS WITH ONION, GARLIC, AND HERBS. THIS QUICK SAUTÉED VERSION—MADE HEARTIER WITH CAULIFLOWER—ACTS AS BOTH RELISH AND SIDE DISH.

- 2 4- to 6-ounce tri-tip steaks, cut ¾ to 1 inch thick
- ¾ teaspoon black pepper
- 2 tablespoons extra virgin olive oil
- 2 red and/or yellow sweet peppers, seeded and sliced
- 1 shallot, thinly sliced
- 1 teaspoon Mediterranean Seasoning (see recipe)
- 2 cups small cauliflower florets
- 2 tablespoons balsamic vinegar
- 2 teaspoons snipped fresh thyme

1. Pat steaks dry with paper towels. Sprinkle steaks with ¼ teaspoon of the black pepper. In a large skillet heat 1 tablespoon of the oil over medium-high heat. Add steaks to skillet; reduce heat to medium. Cook steaks for 6 to 9 minutes for medium rare (145°F), turning occasionally. (If meat browns too quickly, reduce heat.) Remove steaks from skillet; cover loosely with foil to keep warm.

2. For the peperonata, add the remaining 1 tablespoon oil to the skillet. Add the sweet peppers and shallot. Sprinkle with Mediterranean Seasoning. Cook over medium heat about 5 minutes or until peppers are softened, stirring occasionally. Add cauliflower, balsamic vinegar, thyme,

and the remaining ½ teaspoon black pepper. Cover and cook for 10 to 15 minutes or until cauliflower is tender, stirring occasionally. Return steaks to skillet. Spoon peperonata mixture over steaks. Serve immediately.

FLAT-IRON STEAKS AU POIVRE WITH MUSHROOM-DIJON SAUCE

PREP: 15 minutes COOK: 20 minutes MAKES: 4 servings

THIS FRENCH-INSPIRED STEAK WITH MUSHROOM SAUCE CAN BE ON THE TABLE IN JUST OVER 30 MINUTES—WHICH MAKES IT A GREAT CHOICE FOR A QUICK WEEKNIGHT MEAL.

STEAKS
- 3 tablespoons extra virgin olive oil
- 1 pound small asparagus spears, trimmed
- 4 6-ounce flat-iron (boneless beef shoulder top blade) steaks*
- 2 tablespoons snipped fresh rosemary
- 1½ teaspoons cracked black pepper

SAUCE
- 8 ounces sliced fresh mushrooms
- 2 cloves garlic, minced
- ½ cup Beef Bone Broth (see recipe)
- ¼ cup dry white wine
- 1 tablespoon Dijon-Style Mustard (see recipe)

1. In a large skillet heat 1 tablespoon of the oil over medium-high heat. Add asparagus; cook for 8 to 10 minutes or until crisp-tender, turning spears occasionally so they don't burn. Transfer asparagus to a plate; cover with foil to keep warm.

2. Sprinkle steaks with rosemary and pepper; rub in with your fingers. In the same skillet heat the remaining 2 tablespoons oil over medium-high heat. Add steaks; reduce heat to medium. Cook for 8 to 12 minutes for medium rare (145°F), turning meat occasionally. (If meat

browns too quickly, reduce heat.) Remove meat from skillet, reserving drippings. Cover steaks loosely with foil to keep warm.

3. For sauce, add mushrooms and garlic to drippings in skillet; cook until tender, stirring occasionally. Add broth, wine, and Dijon-Style Mustard. Cook over medium heat, scraping up the browned bits in bottom of skillet. Bring to boiling; cook for 1 minute more.

4. Divide the asparagus among four dinner plates. Top with steaks; spoon sauce over the steaks.

*Note: If you can't find 6-ounce flat-iron steaks, purchase two 8- to 12-ounce steaks and cut them in half to make four steaks.

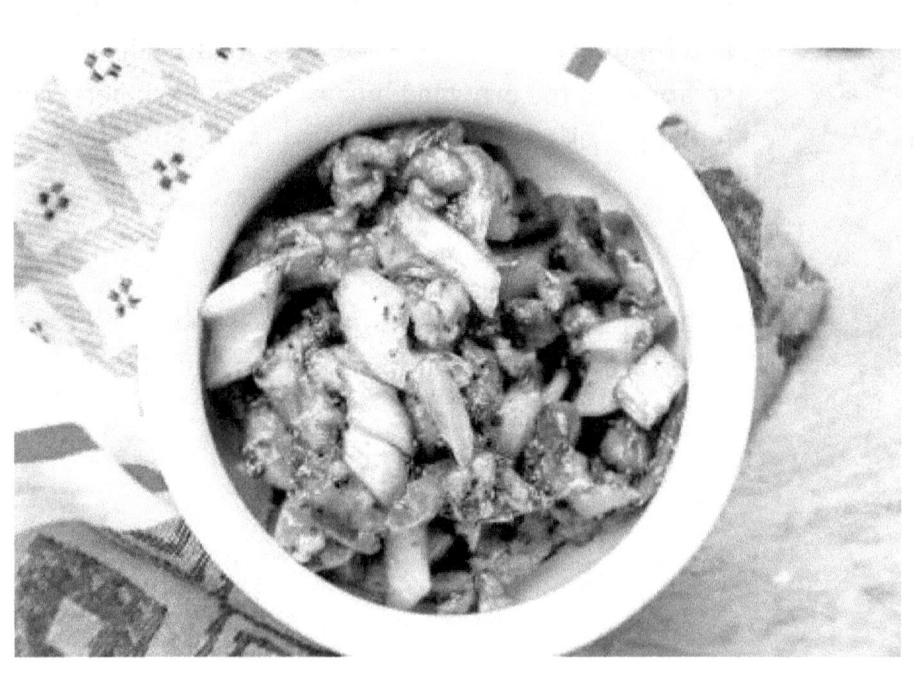

GRILLED FLAT-IRON STEAKS WITH CHIPOTLE-CARAMELIZED ONIONS AND SALSA SALAD

PREP: 30 minutes MARINATE: 2 hours BAKE: 20 minutes COOL: 20 minutes GRILL: 45 minutes MAKES: 4 servings

FLAT-IRON STEAK IS A RELATIVELY NEW CUT DEVELOPED JUST A FEW YEARS AGO. CUT FROM THE FLAVORFUL CHUCK SECTION NEAR THE SHOULDER BLADE, IT IS SURPRISINGLY TENDER AND TASTES MUCH MORE EXPENSIVE THAN IT IS—WHICH LIKELY ACCOUNTS FOR ITS QUICK RISE IN POPULARITY.

STEAKS
⅓ cup fresh lime juice
¼ cup extra virgin olive oil
¼ cup coarsely chopped cilantro
5 cloves garlic, minced
4 6-ounce flat-iron (boneless beef shoulder top blade) steaks

SALSA SALAD
1 seedless (English) cucumber (peeled if desired), diced
1 cup quartered grape tomatoes
½ cup diced red onion
½ cup coarsely chopped cilantro
1 poblano chile, seeded and diced (see tip)
1 jalapeño, seeded and minced (see tip)
3 tablespoons fresh lime juice
2 tablespoons extra virgin olive oil

CARAMELIZED ONIONS
2 tablespoons extra virgin olive oil
2 large sweet onions (such as Maui, Vidalia, Texas Sweet, or Walla Walla)

½ teaspoon ground chipotle chile pepper

1. For steaks, place steaks in a resealable plastic bag set in a shallow dish; set aside. In a small bowl combine lime juice, oil, cilantro, and garlic; pour over steaks in bag. Seal bag; turn to coat. Marinate in the refrigerator for 2 hours.

2. For salad, in a large bowl combine cucumber, tomatoes, onion, cilantro, poblano, and jalapeño. Toss to combine. For dressing, in a small bowl whisk together lime juice and olive oil together. Drizzle dressing over vegetables; toss to coat. Cover and refrigerate until serving time.

3. For onions, preheat oven to 400°F. Brush the inside of a Dutch oven with some of the olive oil; set aside. Cut onions in half lengthwise, remove skins, and then slice crosswise ¼ inch thick. In the Dutch oven combine the remaining olive oil, the onions, and the chipotle chile pepper. Cover and bake for 20 minutes. Uncover and let cool about 20 minutes.

4. Transfer cooled onions to a foil grilling bag or wrap onions in a double thickness of foil. Puncture the top of the foil in several places with a skewer.

5. For a charcoal grill, arrange medium-hot coals around perimeter of grill. Test for medium heat above center of grill. Place packet in center of grill rack. Cover and grill about 45 minutes or until onions are soft and amber color. (For a gas grill, preheat grill. Reduce heat to medium. Adjust for indirect cooking. Place packet over the burner that is turned off. Cover and grill as directed.)

6. Remove steaks from marinade; discard marinade. For a charcoal or gas grill, place steaks on the grill rack directly over medium-high heat. Cover and grill for 8 to 10 minutes or until an instant-read thermometer inserted horizontally into the steaks reads 135°F, turning once. Transfer steaks to a platter, cover loosely with foil and let stand for 10 minutes.

7. To serve, divide salsa salad among four serving plates. Place a steak on each plate and top with a mound of caramelized onions. Serve immediately.

Make-Ahead Directions: Salsa salad may be made and refrigerated up to 4 hours before serving.

GRILLED RIBEYES WITH HERBED ONION AND GARLIC "BUTTER"

PREP: 10 minutes COOK: 12 minutes CHILL: 30 minutes GRILL: 11 minutes MAKES: 4 servings

THE HEAT FROM JUST-OFF-THE-GRILL STEAKS MELTS THE MOUNDS OF CARAMELIZED ONIONS, GARLIC, AND HERBS SUSPENDED IN A RICH-TASTING BLEND OF COCONUT OIL AND OLIVE OIL.

2 tablespoons unrefined coconut oil

1 small onion, halved and cut into very thin slivers (about ¾ cup)

1 clove garlic, very thinly sliced

2 tablespoons extra virgin olive oil

1 tablespoon snipped fresh parsley

2 teaspoons snipped fresh thyme, rosemary, and/or oregano

4 8- to 10-ounce beef ribeye steaks, cut 1 inch thick

½ teaspoon freshly ground black pepper

1. In a medium skillet melt coconut oil over low heat. Add onion; cook for 10 to 15 minutes or until lightly browned, stirring occasionally. Add garlic; cook for 2 to 3 minutes more or until onion is golden brown, stirring occasionally.

2. Transfer onion mixture to a small bowl. Stir in olive oil, parsley, and thyme. Refrigerate, uncovered, for 30 minutes or until mixture is firm enough to mound when scooped, stirring occasionally.

3. Meanwhile, sprinkle steaks with pepper. For a charcoal or gas grill, place steaks on the grill rack directly over medium heat. Cover and grill for 11 to 15 minutes for

medium rare (145°F) or 14 to 18 minutes for medium (160°F), turning once halfway through grilling.

4. To serve, place each steak on a serving plate. Immediately scoop onion mixture evenly onto steaks.

RIBEYE SALAD WITH GRILLED BEETS

PREP: 20 minutes GRILL: 55 minutes STAND: 5 minutes MAKES: 4 servings

THE EARTHY FLAVOR OF BEETS PAIRS BEAUTIFULLY WITH THE SWEETNESS OF THE ORANGES—AND THE TOASTED PECANS ADD A BIT OF CRUNCH TO THIS MAIN-DISH SALAD THAT'S PERFECT FOR EATING OUTDOORS ON A WARM SUMMER NIGHT.

- 1 pound medium golden and/or red beets, scrubbed, trimmed, and cut into wedges
- 1 small onion, cut into thin wedges
- 2 sprigs fresh thyme
- 1 tablespoon extra virgin olive oil
- Cracked black pepper
- 2 8-ounce boneless beef ribeye steaks, cut ¾ inch thick
- 2 cloves garlic, halved
- 2 tablespoons Mediterranean Seasoning (see recipe)
- 6 cups mixed greens
- 2 oranges, peeled, sectioned, and coarsely chopped
- ½ cup chopped pecans, toasted (see tip)
- ½ cup Bright Citrus Vinaigrette (see recipe)

1. Place beets, onion, and thyme sprigs in a foil pan. Drizzle with oil and toss to combine; sprinkle lightly with cracked black pepper. For a charcoal or gas grill, place pan on the center of the grill rack. Cover and grill 55 to 60 minutes or until tender when pierced with a knife, stirring occasionally.

2. Meanwhile, rub both sides of the steaks with cut sides of garlic; sprinkle with Mediterranean Seasoning.

3. Move beets from center of grill to make room for steaks. Add steaks to grill directly over medium heat. Cover and

grill for 11 to 15 minutes for medium rare (145°F) or 14 to 18 minutes for medium (160°F), turning once halfway through grilling. Remove foil pan and steaks from grill. Let steaks stand for 5 minutes. Discard thyme sprigs from foil pan.

4. Thinly slice steak diagonally into bite-size pieces. Divide greens among four serving plates. Top with sliced steak, beets, onion wedges, chopped oranges, and pecans. Drizzle with Bright Citrus Vinaigrette.

KOREAN-STYLE SHORT RIBS WITH SAUTÉED GINGER CABBAGE

PREP: 50 minutes COOK: 25 minutes BAKE: 10 hours CHILL: overnight MAKES: 4 servings

MAKE SURE THE LID OF YOUR DUTCH OVEN FITS VERY TIGHTLY SO THAT DURING THE VERY LONG BRAISING TIME, THE COOKING LIQUID DOESN'T ALL EVAPORATE THROUGH A GAP BETWEEN THE LID AND POT.

1 ounce dried shiitake mushrooms
1½ cups sliced scallions
1 Asian pear, peeled, cored, and chopped
1 3-inch piece fresh ginger, peeled and chopped
1 serrano chile pepper, finely chopped (seeded if desired) (see tip)
5 cloves garlic
1 tablespoon refined coconut oil
5 pounds bone-in beef short ribs
Freshly ground black pepper
4 cups Beef Bone Broth (see recipe) or no-salt-added beef broth
2 cups sliced fresh shiitake mushrooms
1 tablespoon finely shredded orange peel
⅓ cup fresh juice
Sautéed Ginger Cabbage (see recipe, below)
Finely shredded orange peel (optional)

1. Preheat oven to 325°F. Place dried shiitake mushrooms in a small bowl; add enough boiling water to cover. Let stand about 30 minutes or until rehydrated and soft. Drain, reserving the soaking liquid. Finely chop the mushrooms. Place mushrooms in a small bowl; cover and refrigerate until needed in Step 4. Set mushrooms and liquid aside.

2. For sauce, in a food processor combine scallions, Asian pear, ginger, serrano, garlic, and the reserved mushroom soaking liquid. Cover and process until smooth. Set sauce aside.

3. In a 6-quart Dutch oven heat the coconut oil over medium-high heat. Sprinkle short ribs with freshly ground black pepper. Cook ribs, in batches, in hot coconut oil about 10 minutes or until well browned on all sides, turning halfway through cooking. Return all the ribs to the pot; add sauce and Beef Bone broth. Cover the Dutch oven with a tight-fitting lid. Bake about 10 hours or until meat is very tender and falls off the bones.

4. Carefully remove the ribs from sauce. Place ribs and sauce in separate containers. Cover and refrigerate overnight. When cold, remove fat from surface of the sauce and discard. Bring the sauce to boiling over high heat; add hydrated mushrooms from Step 1 and the fresh mushrooms. Boil gently for 10 minutes to reduce sauce and intensify flavors. Return ribs to the sauce; simmer until heated through. Stir in 1 tablespoon orange peel and the orange juice. Serve with Sautéed Ginger Cabbage. If desired, sprinkle with additional orange peel.

Sautéed Ginger Cabbage: In a large skillet heat 1 tablespoon refined coconut oil over medium-high heat. Add 2 tablespoons minced fresh ginger; 2 cloves garlic, minced; and crushed red pepper to taste. Cook and stir until fragrant, about 30 seconds. Add 6 cups shredded napa, savoy, or green cabbage and 1 Asian pear, peeled, cored, and thinly sliced. Cook and stir for 3 minutes or until cabbage wilts slightly and pear softens. Stir in ½ cup unsweetened apple juice. Cover and cook about 2 minutes until cabbage is tender. Stir in ½ cup sliced scallions and 1 tablespoon sesame seeds.

BEEF SHORT RIBS WITH CITRUS-FENNEL GREMOLATA

PREP: 40 minutes GRILL: 8 minutes SLOW COOK: 9 hours (low) or 4½ hours (high) MAKES: 4 servings

GREMOLATA IS A FLAVORFUL BLEND OF PARSLEY, GARLIC, AND LEMON PEEL THAT IS SPRINKLED ON OSSO BUCCO—THE CLASSIC ITALIAN DISH OF BRAISED VEAL SHANKS—TO BRIGHTEN ITS RICH, UNCTUOUS FLAVOR. WITH THE ADDITION OF ORANGE PEEL AND FRESH FEATHERY FENNEL FRONDS, IT DOES THE SAME FOR THESE TENDER BEEF SHORT RIBS.

RIBS
- 2½ to 3 pounds bone-in beef short ribs
- 3 tablespoons Lemon-Herb Seasoning (see recipe)
- 1 medium fennel bulb
- 1 large onion, cut into large wedges
- 2 cups Beef Bone Broth (see recipe) or no-salt-added beef broth
- 2 cloves garlic, halved

PAN-ROASTED SQUASH
- 3 tablespoons extra virgin olive oil
- 1 pound butternut squash, peeled, seeded, and cut into ½-inch pieces (about 2 cups)
- 4 teaspoons snipped fresh thyme
- Extra virgin olive oil

GREMOLATA
- ¼ cup snipped fresh parsley
- 2 tablespoons minced garlic
- 1½ teaspoons finely shredded lemon peel
- 1½ teaspoons finely shredded orange peel

1. Sprinkle short ribs with Lemon-Herb Seasoning; lightly rub into meat with your fingers; set aside. Remove fronds from fennel; set aside for Citrus-Fennel Gremolata. Trim and quarter fennel bulb.

2. For a charcoal grill, arrange medium-hot coals on one side of the grill. Test for medium heat above the side of grill without coals. Place short ribs on grill rack on side without coals; place fennel quarters and onion wedges on the rack directly over coals. Cover and grill for 8 to 10 minutes or until vegetables and ribs are just browned, turning once halfway through grilling. (For a gas grill, preheat grill, reduce heat to medium. Adjust for indirect cooking. Place ribs on grill rack over burner that is turned off; place fennel and onion on rack over burner that is turned on. Cover and grill as directed.) When cool enough to handle, coarsely chop the fennel and onion.

3. In a 5- to 6-quart slow cooker combine chopped fennel and onion, Beef Bone Broth, and garlic. Add ribs. Cover and cook on low-heat setting for 9 to 10 hours or 4½ to 5 hours on high-heat setting. Using a slotted spoon, transfer ribs to a platter; cover with foil to keep warm.

4. Meanwhile, for the squash, in a large skillet heat the 3 tablespoons oil over medium-high heat. Add squash and 3 teaspoons of the thyme, stirring to coat the squash. Arrange squash in a single layer in skillet and cook without stirring about 3 minutes or until browned on bottom sides. Turn squash pieces over; cook about 3 minutes more or until second sides are browned. Reduce heat to low; cover and cook for 10 to 15 minutes or until

tender. Sprinkle with remaining 1 teaspoon fresh thyme; drizzle with additional extra virgin olive oil.

5. For the gremolata, finely chop enough reserved fennel fronds to make ¼ cup. In a small bowl stir together the chopped fennel fronds, parsley, garlic, lemon peel, and orange peel.

6. Sprinkle gremolata over ribs. Serve with squash.

SWEDISH-STYLE BEEF PATTIES WITH MUSTARD-DILL CUCUMBER SALAD

PREP: 30 minutes COOK: 15 minutes MAKES: 4 servings

BEEF À LA LINDSTROM IS A SWEDISH HAMBURGER THAT IS TRADITIONALLY STUDDED WITH ONIONS, CAPERS, AND PICKLED BEETS SERVED WITH GRAVY AND WITHOUT A BUN. THIS ALLSPICE-INFUSED VERSION SUBSTITUTES ROASTED BEETS FOR THE SALT-LADEN PICKLED BEETS AND CAPERS AND IS TOPPED WITH A FRIED EGG.

CUCUMBER SALAD
- 2 teaspoons fresh orange juice
- 2 teaspoons white wine vinegar
- 1 teaspoon Dijon-Style Mustard (see recipe)
- 1 tablespoon extra virgin olive oil
- 1 large seedless (English) cucumber, peeled and sliced
- 2 tablespoons sliced scallions
- 1 tablespoon chopped fresh dill

BEEF PATTIES
- 1 pound ground beef
- ¼ cup finely chopped onion
- 1 tablespoon Dijon-Style Mustard (see recipe)
- ¾ teaspoon black pepper
- ½ teaspoon ground allspice
- ½ of a small beet, roasted, peeled, and finely diced*
- 2 tablespoons extra virgin olive oil
- ½ cup Beef Bone Broth (see recipe) or no-salt-added beef broth
- 4 large eggs
- 1 tablespoon finely chopped chives

1. For cucumber salad, in a large bowl whisk together orange juice, vinegar, and Dijon-Style Mustard. Slowly add olive oil in a thin stream, whisking until dressing thickens slightly. Add cucumber, scallions, and dill; toss until combined. Cover and refrigerate until serving time.

2. For beef patties, in a large bowl combine ground beef, onion, Dijon-Style Mustard, pepper, and allspice. Add roasted beet and gently mix until evenly incorporated into the meat. Shape mixture into four ½-inch-thick patties.

3. In a large skillet heat 1 tablespoon olive oil over medium-high heat. Fry patties about 8 minutes or until browned on the exterior and cooked through (160°), turning once. Transfer patties to a plate and cover loosely with foil to keep warm. Add Beef Bone Broth, stirring to scrape up browned bits from bottom of skillet. Cook about 4 minutes or until reduced by half. Drizzle patties with reduced pan juices and re-cover loosely.

4. Rinse and wipe out skillet with a paper towel. Heat the remaining 1 tablespoon olive oil over medium heat. Fry eggs in hot oil for 3 to 4 minutes or until whites are cooked but yolks remain soft and runny.

5. Place an egg on each beef patty. Sprinkle with chives and serve with cucumber salad.

*Tip: To roast beet, scrub well and place on a piece of aluminum foil. Drizzle with a little olive oil. Wrap in foil and seal tightly. Roast in a 375°F oven about 30 minutes or until a fork easily pierces beet. Let cool; slip skin off.

(Beet can be roasted up to 3 days ahead. Tightly wrap peeled roasted beets and store in the refrigerator.)

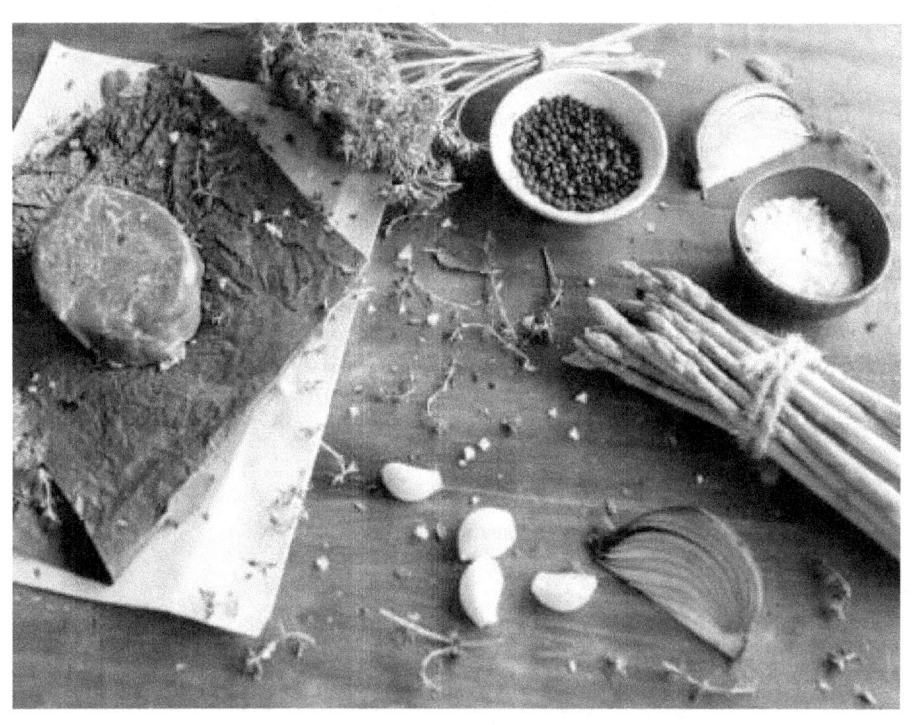

SMOTHERED BEEFBURGERS ON ARUGULA WITH ROASTED ROOT VEGETABLES

PREP: 40 minutes COOK: 35 minutes ROAST: 20 minutes MAKES: 4 servings

THERE ARE A LOT OF ELEMENTS TO THESE HEARTY BURGERS—AND THEY DO TAKE A BIT OF TIME TO PUT TOGETHER—BUT THE INCREDIBLE COMBINATION OF FLAVORS MAKES IT WELL WORTH THE EFFORT: A MEATY BURGER IS TOPPED WITH CARAMELIZED ONION AND MUSHROOM PAN SAUCE AND SERVED WITH SWEET ROASTED VEGETABLES AND PEPPERY ARUGULA.

- 5 tablespoons extra virgin olive oil
- 2 cups sliced fresh button, cremini, and/or shiitake mushrooms
- 3 yellow onions, thinly sliced*
- 2 teaspoons caraway seeds
- 3 carrots, peeled and cut into 1-inch chunks
- 2 parsnips, peeled and cut into 1-inch chunks
- 1 acorn squash, halved, seeded, and cut into wedges
- Freshly ground black pepper
- 2 pounds ground beef
- ½ cup finely chopped onion
- 1 tablespoon salt-free all-purpose seasoning blend
- 2 cups Beef Bone Broth (see [recipe](#)) or no-salt-added beef broth
- ¼ cup unsweetened apple juice
- 1 to 2 tablespoons dry sherry or white wine vinegar
- 1 tablespoon Dijon-Style Mustard (see [recipe](#))
- 1 tablespoon snipped fresh thyme leaves
- 1 tablespoon snipped fresh parsley leaves
- 8 cups arugula leaves

1. Preheat oven to 425°F. For sauce, in a large skillet heat 1 tablespoon of the olive oil over medium-high heat. Add mushrooms; cook and stir about 8 minutes or until well browned and tender. Using a slotted spoon, transfer the mushrooms to a plate. Return the skillet to the burner; reduce heat to medium. Add the remaining 1 tablespoon olive oil, sliced onions, and the caraway seeds. Cover and cook for 20 to 25 minutes or until onions are very soft and richly browned, stirring occasionally. (Adjust heat as needed to prevent the onions from burning.)

2. Meanwhile, for roasted root vegetables, on a large baking sheet arrange carrots, parsnips, and squash. Drizzle with 2 tablespoons olive oil and sprinkle with pepper to taste; toss to coat vegetables. Roast for 20 to 25 minutes or until tender and beginning to brown, turning once halfway through roasting. Keep vegetables warm until ready to serve.

3. For burgers, in a large bowl combine the ground beef, finely chopped onion, and seasoning blend. Divide meat mixture into four equal portions and shape into patties, about ¾ inch thick. In an extra-large skillet heat the remaining 1 tablespoon olive oil over medium-high heat. Add burgers to skillet; cook about 8 minutes or until seared on both sides, turning once. Transfer burgers to a plate.

4. Add caramelized onions, reserved mushrooms, Beef Bone Broth, apple juice, sherry, and Dijon-Style Mustard to the skillet, stirring to combine. Return burgers to skillet. Bring to simmering. Cook until burgers are done (160°F), about

7 to 8 minutes. Stir in fresh thyme, parsley, and pepper to taste.

5. To serve, arrange 2 cups of arugula on each of four serving plates. Divide the roasted vegetables among the salads, then top with burgers. Generously spoon the onion mixture on the burgers.

*Tip: A mandoline slicer is a great help in thinly slicing onions.

GRILLED BEEFBURGERS WITH SESAME-CRUSTED TOMATOES

PREP: 30 minutes STAND: 20 minutes GRILL: 10 minutes MAKES: 4 servings

CRISP, GOLDEN-BROWN SESAME-CRUSTED SLICES OF TOMATO STAND IN FOR THE TRADITIONAL SESAME SEED BUN IN THESE SMOKY BURGERS. SERVE THEM WITH A KNIFE AND FORK.

4 ½-inch-thick red or green tomato slices*
1¼ pounds lean ground beef
1 tablespoon Smoky Seasoning (see recipe)
1 large egg
¾ cup almond meal
¼ cup sesame seeds
¼ teaspoon black pepper
1 small red onion, halved and sliced
1 tablespoon extra virgin olive oil
¼ cup refined coconut oil
1 small head Bibb lettuce
Paleo Ketchup (see recipe)
Dijon-Style Mustard (see recipe)

1. Place tomato slices on a double layer of paper towels. Top tomatoes with another double layer of paper towels. Press down lightly on paper towels so they stick to the tomatoes. Let stand at room temperature for 20 to 30 minutes so some of the tomato juice is absorbed.

2. Meanwhile, in a large bowl combine ground beef and Smoky Seasoning. Shape into four ½-inch-thick patties.

3. In a shallow bowl lightly beat egg with a fork. In another shallow bowl combine almond meal, sesame seeds, and

pepper. Dip each tomato slice into the egg, turning to coat. Allow excess egg to drip off. Dip each tomato slice into almond meal mixture, turning to coat. Place coated tomatoes on a flat plate; set aside. Toss onion slices with olive oil; place onion slices in a grill basket.

4. For a charcoal or gas grill, place onions in basket and beef patties on grill rack over medium heat. Cover and grill for 10 to 12 minutes or onions are golden brown and lightly charred and patties are done (160°), stirring onions occasionally and turning patties once.

5. Meanwhile, in a large skillet heat oil over medium heat. Add tomato slices; cook for 8 to 10 minutes or until golden brown, turning once. (If tomatoes brown too quickly, reduce heat to medium-low. If necessary, add additional oil.) Drain on a paper towel-lined plate.

6. To serve, divide lettuce among four serving plates. Top with patties, onions, Paleo Ketchup, Dijon-Style Mustard, and sesame-crusted tomatoes.

*Note: You'll probably need 2 large tomatoes. If using red tomatoes, choose tomatoes that are just ripe but still slightly firm.

BURGERS ON A STICK WITH BABA GHANOUSH DIPPING SAUCE

SOAK: 15 minutes PREP: 20 minutes GRILL: 35 minutes MAKES: 4 servings

BABA GHANOUSH IS A MIDDLE EASTERN SPREAD MADE FROM SMOKY GRILLED EGGPLANT PUREED WITH OLIVE OIL, LEMON, GARLIC, AND TAHINI, A PASTE MADE FROM GROUND SESAME SEEDS. A SPRINKLING OF SESAME SEEDS IS FINE, BUT WHEN THEY ARE MADE INTO OIL OR PASTE, THEY BECOME A CONCENTRATED SOURCE OF LINOLEIC ACID, WHICH CAN CONTRIBUTE TO INFLAMMATION. THE PINE NUT BUTTER USED HERE MAKES A FINE SUBSTITUTE.

- 4 dried tomatoes
- 1½ pounds lean ground beef
- 3 to 4 tablespoons finely chopped onion
- 1 tablespoon finely snipped fresh oregano and/or finely snipped fresh mint or ½ teaspoon dried oregano, crushed
- ¼ teaspoon cayenne pepper
- Baba Ghanoush Dipping Sauce (see recipe, below)

1. Soak eight 10-inch wooden skewers in water for 30 minutes. Meanwhile, in a small bowl pour boiling water over tomatoes; let stand for 5 minutes to rehydrate. Drain tomatoes and pat dry with paper towels.

2. In large bowl combine chopped tomatoes, ground beef, onion, oregano, and cayenne pepper. Divide meat mixture into eight portions; roll each portion into a ball. Remove skewers from water; pat dry. Thread one ball onto a skewer and shape into a long oval around the skewer, starting just below the pointed tip and leaving enough

room on the other end to be able to hold the stick. Repeat with remaining skewers and balls.

3. For a charcoal or gas grill, place beef skewers on a grill rack directly over medium heat. Cover and grill about 6 minutes or until done (160°F), turning once halfway through grilling. Serve with Baba Ghanoush Dipping Sauce.

Baba Ghanoush Dipping Sauce: Poke 2 medium eggplants in several places with a fork. For a charcoal or gas grill, place eggplants on a grill rack directly over medium heat. Cover and grill for 10 minutes or until charred on all sides, turning several times during grilling. Remove eggplants and carefully wrap in foil. Place wrapped eggplants back on the grill rack but not directly over the coals. Cover and grill for 25 to 35 minutes more or until collapsed and very tender. Cool. Halve eggplants and scrape out the flesh; place flesh in a food processor. Add ¼ cup Pine Nut Butter (see recipe); ¼ cup fresh lemon juice; 2 cloves garlic, minced; 1 tablespoon extra virgin olive oil; 2 to 3 tablespoons snipped fresh parsley; and ½ teaspoon ground cumin. Cover and process just until almost smooth. If sauce is too thick for dipping, stir in enough water to make desired consistency.

SMOKY STUFFED SWEET PEPPERS

PREP: 20 minutes COOK: 8 minutes BAKE: 30 minutes MAKES: 4 servings

MAKE THIS FAMILY FAVORITE WITH A MIX OF COLORED SWEET PEPPERS FOR AN EYE-CATCHING DISH. THE FIRE-ROASTED TOMATOES ARE A FINE EXAMPLE OF HOW TO ADD GREAT TASTE TO FOOD IN A HEALTHY WAY. THE SIMPLE ACT OF SLIGHTLY CHARRING THE TOMATOES BEFORE THEY ARE CANNED (WITHOUT SALT) BUMPS UP THEIR FLAVOR.

4 large green, red, yellow, and/or orange sweet peppers
1 pound ground beef
1 tablespoon Smoky Seasoning (see recipe)
1 tablespoon extra virgin olive oil
1 small yellow onion, chopped
3 cloves garlic, minced
1 small head cauliflower, cored and broken into florets
1 15-ounce can no-salt-added diced fire-roasted tomatoes, drained
¼ cup finely chopped fresh parsley
½ teaspoon black pepper
⅛ teaspoon cayenne pepper
½ cup Walnut Crumb Topping (see recipe, below)

1. Preheat oven to 375°F. Cut sweet peppers in half vertically. Remove stems, seeds, and membranes; discard. Set pepper halves aside.

2. Place ground beef in a medium bowl; sprinkle with Smoky Seasoning. Use your hands to gently mix seasoning into meat.

3. In a large skillet heat olive oil over medium heat. Add meat, onion, and garlic; cook until meat is browned and onion is

tender, stirring with a wooden spoon to break up meat. Remove skillet from heat.

4. In a food processor process cauliflower florets until very finely chopped. (If you don't have a food processor, grate the cauliflower on a box grater.) Measure 3 cups of the cauliflower. Add to ground beef mixture in skillet. (If there is any remaining cauliflower, save it for another use.) Stir in drained tomatoes, parsley, black pepper, and cayenne pepper.

5. Fill pepper halves with ground beef mixture, packing it lightly and mounding slightly. Arrange filled pepper halves in a baking dish. Bake for 30 to 35 minutes or until peppers are crisp-tender.* Top with Walnut Crumb Topping. If desired, return to oven for 5 minutes to crisp topping before serving.

Walnut Crumb Topping: In a medium skillet heat 1 tablespoon extra virgin olive oil over medium low heat. Stir in 1 teaspoon dried thyme, 1 teaspoon smoked paprika, and ¼ teaspoon garlic powder. Add 1 cup very finely chopped walnuts. Cook and stir about 5 minutes or until walnuts are golden brown and lightly toasted. Stir in a dash or two of cayenne pepper. Let cool completely. Store leftover topping in a tightly sealed container in the refrigerator until ready to use. Makes 1 cup.

*Note: If using green peppers, bake for an additional 10 minutes.

BISON BURGERS WITH CABERNET ONIONS AND ARUGULA

PREP: 30 minutes COOK: 18 minutes GRILL: 10 minutes MAKES: 4 servings

BISON HAS A VERY LOW FAT CONTENT AND WILL COOK 30% TO 50% FASTER THAN BEEF. THE MEAT RETAINS ITS RED COLOR AFTER COOKING, SO COLOR IS NOT AN INDICATOR OF DONENESS. BECAUSE BISON IS SO LEAN, DO NOT COOK IT BEYOND AN INTERNAL TEMPERATURE OF 155°F.

- 2 tablespoons extra virgin olive oil
- 2 large sweet onions, thinly sliced
- ¾ cup Cabernet Sauvignon or other dry red wine
- 1 teaspoon Mediterranean Seasoning (see recipe)
- ¼ cup extra virgin olive oil
- ¼ cup balsamic vinegar
- 1 tablespoon finely chopped shallot
- 1 tablespoon snipped fresh basil
- 1 small clove garlic, minced
- 1 pound ground bison
- ¼ cup Basil Pesto (see recipe)
- 5 cups arugula
- Raw unsalted pistachios, toasted (see tip)

1. In a large skillet heat the 2 tablespoons oil over medium-low heat. Add onions. Cook, covered, for 10 to 15 minutes or until onions are tender, stirring occasionally. Uncover; cook and stir over medium-high heat for 3 to 5 minutes or until onions are golden. Add wine; cook about 5 minutes or until most of the wine evaporates. Sprinkle with Mediterranean Seasoning; keep warm.

2. Meanwhile, for vinaigrette, in a screw-top jar combine the ¼ cup olive oil, vinegar, shallot, basil, and garlic. Cover and shake well.

3. In a large bowl lightly mix ground bison and Basil Pesto. Lightly shape meat mixture into four ¾-inch-thick patties.

4. For a charcoal or gas grill, place patties on a lightly greased grill rack directly over medium heat. Cover and grill about 10 minutes to desired doneness (145°F for medium rare or 155°F for medium), turning once halfway through grilling.

5. Place arugula in a large bowl. Drizzle vinaigrette over arugula; toss to coat. To serve, divide onions among four serving plates; top each with a bison burger. Top burgers with arugula and sprinkle with pistachios.

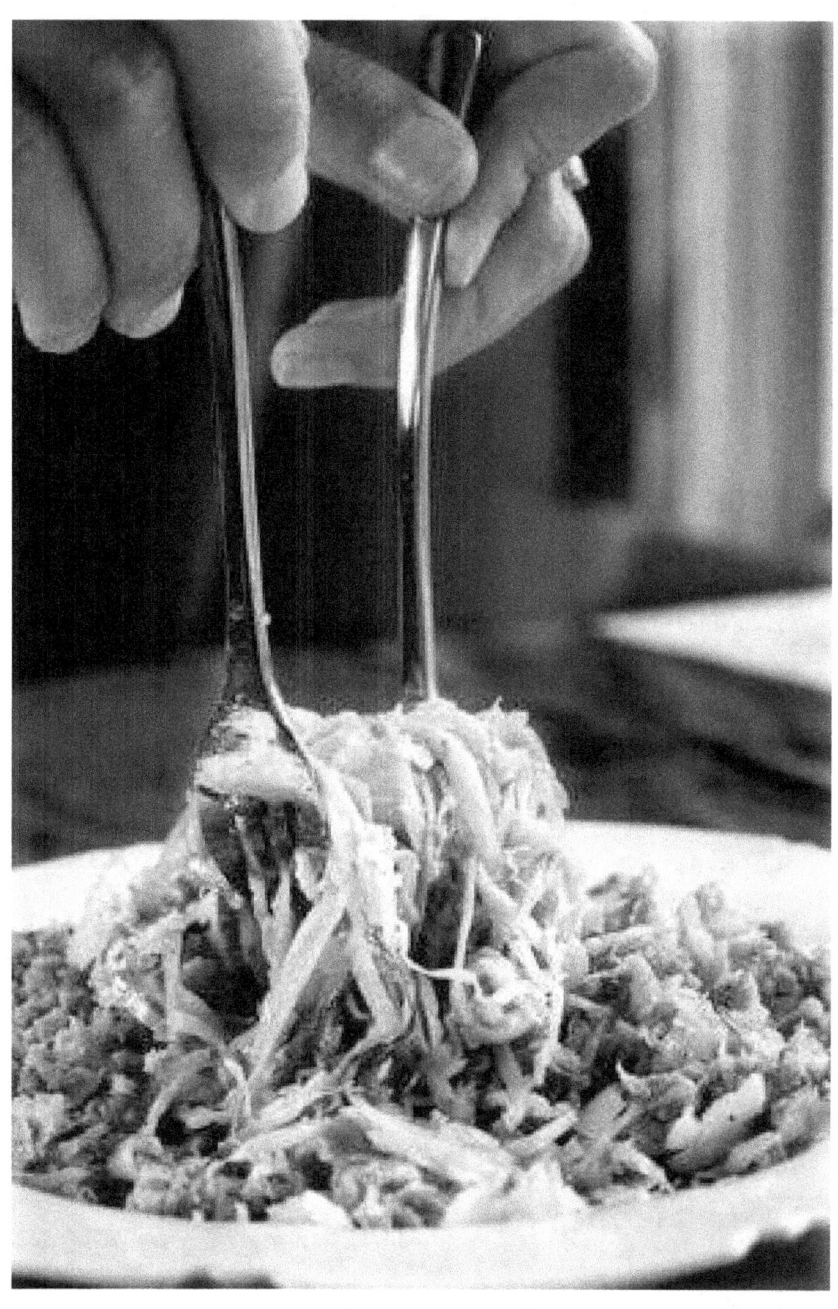

BISON AND LAMB MEAT LOAF ON CHARD AND SWEET POTATOES

PREP: 1 hour COOK: 20 minutes BAKE: 1 hour STAND: 10 minutes MAKES: 4 servings

THIS IS OLD-FASHIONED COMFORT FOOD WITH A MODERN TWIST. A RED-WINE PAN SAUCE GIVES THE MEAT LOAF A FLAVOR BOOST, AND THE GARLICKY CHARD AND SWEET POTATOES MASHED WITH CASHEW CREAM AND COCONUT OIL OFFER INCREDIBLE NUTRITIONAL CONTENT.

- 2 tablespoons olive oil
- 1 cup finely chopped cremini mushrooms
- ½ cup finely chopped red onion (1 medium)
- ½ cup finely chopped celery (1 stalk)
- ⅓ cup finely chopped carrot (1 small)
- ½ of a small apple, cored, peeled, and shredded
- 2 cloves garlic, minced
- ½ teaspoon Mediterranean Seasoning (see recipe)
- 1 large egg, lightly beaten
- 1 tablespoon snipped fresh sage
- 1 tablespoon snipped fresh thyme
- 8 ounces ground bison
- 8 ounces ground lamb or beef
- ¾ cup dry red wine
- 1 medium shallot, finely chopped
- ¾ cup Beef Bone Broth (see recipe) or no-salt-added beef broth
- Mashed Sweet Potatoes (see recipe, below)
- Garlicky Swiss Chard (see recipe, below)

1. Preheat oven to 350°F. In a large skillet heat oil over medium heat. Add mushrooms, onion, celery, and carrot; cook and stir about 5 minutes or until vegetables are

softened. Reduce heat to low; add shredded apple and garlic. Cook, covered, about 5 minutes or until vegetables are very tender. Remove from heat; stir in Mediterranean Seasoning.

2. Using a slotted spoon, transfer mushroom mixture to a large bowl, reserving drippings in skillet. Stir in egg, sage, and thyme. Add ground bison and ground lamb; lightly mix. Spoon meat mixture into a 2-quart rectangular baking dish; shape into a 7×4-inch rectangle. Bake about 1 hour or until an instant-read thermometer registers 155°F. Let stand for 10 minutes. Carefully remove meat loaf to a serving platter. Cover and keep warm.

3. For the pan sauce, scrape drippings and crusty browned bits from the baking dish into reserved drippings in the skillet. Add wine and shallot. Bring to boiling over medium heat; cook until reduced by half. Add Beef Bone Broth; cook and stir until reduced by half. Remove skillet from heat.

4. To serve, divide Mashed Sweet Potatoes among four serving plates; top with some of the Garlicky Swiss Chard. Slice meat loaf; place slices on Garlicky Swiss Chard and drizzle with the pan sauce.

Mashed Sweet Potatoes: Peel and coarsely chop 4 medium sweet potatoes. In a large saucepan cook potatoes in enough boiling water to cover for 15 minutes or until tender; drain. Mash with a potato masher. Add ½ cup Cashew Cream (see recipe) and 2 tablespoons unrefined coconut oil; mash until smooth. Keep warm.

Garlicky Swiss Chard: Remove stems from 2 bunches Swiss chard and discard. Coarsely chop leaves. In a large skillet heat 2 tablespoons olive oil over medium heat. Add Swiss chard and 2 cloves garlic, minced; cook until chard is wilted, tossing occasionally with tongs.

APPLE-CURRANT-SAUCED BISON MEATBALLS WITH ZUCCHINI PAPPARDELLE

PREP: 25 minutes BAKE: 15 minutes COOK: 18 minutes MAKES: 4 servings

THE MEATBALLS WILL BE VERY WET AS YOU FORM THEM. TO KEEP THE MEAT MIXTURE FROM STICKING TO YOUR HANDS, KEEP A BOWL OF COOL WATER HANDY AND WET YOUR HANDS OCCASIONALLY AS YOU WORK. CHANGE THE WATER A COUPLE OF TIMES AS YOU MAKE THE MEATBALLS.

MEATBALLS
- Olive oil
- ½ cup coarsely chopped red onion
- 2 cloves garlic, minced
- 1 egg, lightly beaten
- ½ cup finely chopped button mushrooms and stems
- 2 tablespoon snipped fresh Italian (flat-leaf) parsley
- 2 teaspoons olive oil
- 1 pound ground bison (coarse ground if available)

APPLE-CURRANT SAUCE
- 2 tablespoons olive oil
- 2 large Granny Smith apples, peeled, cored, and finely chopped
- 2 shallots, minced
- 2 tablespoons fresh lemon juice
- ½ cup Chicken Bone Broth (see recipe) or no-salt-added chicken broth
- 2 to 3 tablespoons dried currants

ZUCCHINI PAPPARDELLE
- 6 zucchini
- 2 tablespoons olive oil

¼ cup finely chopped scallions

½ teaspoon crushed red pepper

2 cloves garlic, minced

1. For meatballs, preheat oven to 375°F. Lightly brush a rimmed baking sheet with olive oil; set aside. In a food processor or blender combine onion and garlic. Pulse until smooth. Transfer onion mixture to a medium bowl. Add egg, mushrooms, parsley, and 2 teaspoons oil; stir to combine. Add ground bison; mix lightly but well. Divide meat mixture into 16 portions; shape into meatballs. Place meatballs, evenly spaced, on the prepared baking sheet. Bake for 15 minutes; set aside.

2. For sauce, in a skillet heat 2 tablespoons oil over medium heat. Add apples and shallots; cook and stir for 6 to 8 minutes or until very tender. Stir in lemon juice. Transfer mixture to a food processor or blender. Cover and process or blend until smooth; return to the skillet. Stir in Chicken Bone Broth and currants. Bring to boiling; reduce heat. Simmer, uncovered, for 8 to 10 minutes, stirring frequently. Add meatballs; cook and stir over low heat until heated through.

3. Meanwhile, for pappardelle, trim ends of zucchini. Using a mandoline or very sharp vegetable peeler, shave zucchini into thin ribbons. (To keep the ribbons intact, stop shaving once you reach the seeds in the center of the squash.) In a extra-large skillet heat 2 tablespoons oil over medium heat. Stir in scallions, crushed red pepper, and garlic; cook and stir for 30 seconds. Add zucchini ribbons. Cook and gently stir about 3 minutes or just until wilted.

4. To serve, divide pappardelle among four serving plates; top with meatballs and apple-currant sauce.

BISON-PORCINI BOLOGNESE WITH ROASTED GARLIC SPAGHETTI SQUASH

PREP: 30 minutes COOK: 1 hour 30 minutes BAKE: 35 minutes MAKES: 6 servings

IF YOU THOUGHT YOU'D EATEN YOUR LAST DISH OF SPAGHETTI WITH MEAT SAUCE WHEN YOU ADOPTED THE PALEO DIET®, THINK AGAIN. THIS RICH BOLOGNESE FLAVORED WITH GARLIC, RED WINE, AND EARTHY PORCINI MUSHROOMS IS LADELED OVER SWEET, TOOTHSOME STRANDS OF SPAGHETTI SQUASH. YOU WON'T MISS THE PASTA ONE BIT.

- 1 ounce dried porcini mushrooms
- 1 cup boiling water
- 3 tablespoons extra virgin olive oil
- 1 pound ground bison
- 1 cup finely chopped carrots (2)
- ½ cup chopped onion (1 medium)
- ½ cup finely chopped celery (1 stalk)
- 4 cloves garlic, minced
- 3 tablespoons salt-free tomato paste
- ½ cup red wine
- 2 15-ounce cans no-salt-added crushed tomatoes
- 1 teaspoon dried oregano, crushed
- 1 teaspoon dried thyme, crushed
- ½ teaspoon black pepper
- 1 medium spaghetti squash (2½ to 3 pounds)
- 1 bulb garlic

1. In a small bowl combine the porcini mushrooms and boiling water; let stand for 15 minutes. Strain through a sieve lined with 100%-cotton cheesecloth, reserving the soaking liquid. Chop the mushrooms; set side.

2. In a 4- to 5-quart Dutch oven heat 1 tablespoon of the olive oil over medium heat. Add ground bison, carrots, onion, celery, and garlic. Cook until meat is browned and vegetables are tender, stirring with a wooden spoon to break up meat. Add tomato paste; cook and stir for 1 minute. Add red wine; cook and stir for 1 minute. Stir in porcini mushrooms, tomatoes, oregano, thyme, and pepper. Add reserved mushroom liquid, being careful to avoid adding any sand or grit that may be present in the bottom of the bowl. Bring to boiling, stirring occasionally; reduce heat to low. Simmer, covered, for 1½ to 2 hours or until desired consistency.

3. Meanwhile, preheat oven to 375°F. Halve squash lengthwise; scrape out seeds. Place squash halves, cut sides down, in a large baking dish. Using a fork, prick the skin all over. Cut off the top ½ inch of the head of garlic. Place the garlic, cut end up, in the baking dish with the squash. Drizzle with the remaining 1 tablespoon olive oil. Bake for 35 to 45 minutes or until squash and garlic are tender.

4. Using a spoon and fork, remove and shred the squash flesh from each squash half; transfer to a bowl and cover to keep warm. When the garlic is cool enough to handle, squeeze the bulb from the bottom to pop out the cloves. Use a fork to mash the garlic cloves. Stir mashed garlic into the squash, distributing garlic evenly. To serve, spoon sauce over squash mixture.

BISON CHILI CON CARNE

PREP: 25 minutes COOK: 1 hour 10 minutes MAKES: 4 servings

UNSWEETENED CHOCOLATE, COFFEE, AND CINNAMON ADD INTEREST TO THIS HEARTY FAVORITE. IF YOU'D LIKE EVEN MORE SMOKY FLAVOR, SUBSTITUTE 1 TABLESPOON OF SWEET SMOKED PAPRIKA FOR THE REGULAR PAPRIKA.

- 3 tablespoons extra virgin olive oil
- 1 pound ground bison
- ½ cup chopped onion (1 medium)
- 2 cloves garlic, minced
- 2 14.5-ounce cans diced no-salt-added tomatoes, undrained
- 1 6-ounce can salt-free tomato paste
- 1 cup Beef Bone Broth (see recipe) or no-salt-added beef broth
- ½ cup strong coffee
- 2 ounces 99% cacao baking bar, chopped
- 1 tablespoon paprika
- 1 teaspoon ground cumin
- 1 teaspoon dried oregano
- 1½ teaspoons Smoky Seasoning (see recipe)
- ½ teaspoon ground cinnamon
- ⅓ cup pepitas
- 1 teaspoon olive oil
- ½ cup Cashew Cream (see recipe)
- 1 teaspoon fresh lime juice
- ½ cup fresh cilantro leaves
- 4 lime wedges

1. In a Dutch oven heat the 3 tablespoons olive oil over medium heat. Add ground bison, onion, and garlic; cook about 5 minutes or until meat is browned, stirring with a wooden spoon to break up meat. Stir in undrained

tomatoes, tomato paste, Beef Bone Broth, coffee, baking chocolate, paprika, cumin, oregano, 1 teaspoon of the Smoky Seasoning, and cinnamon. Bring to boiling; reduce heat. Simmer, covered, for 1 hour, stirring occasionally.

2. Meanwhile, in a small skillet toast pepitas in the 1 teaspoon olive oil over medium heat until they start to pop and turn golden. Place pepitas in a small bowl; add the remaining ½ teaspoon Smoky Seasoning; toss to coat.

3. In a small bowl combine Cashew Cream and lime juice.

4. To serve, ladle chili into bowls. Top servings with Cashew Cream, pepitas, and cilantro. Serve with lime wedges.

MOROCCAN-SPICED BISON STEAKS WITH GRILLED LEMONS

PREP: 10 minutes GRILL: 10 minutes MAKES: 4 servings

SERVE THESE QUICK-TO-FIX STEAKS WITH COOL AND CRISP SPICED CARROT SLAW (SEE RECIPE). IF YOU'RE CRAVING A TREAT, GRILLED PINEAPPLE WITH COCONUT CREAM (SEE RECIPE) WOULD BE A GREAT WAY TO END THE MEAL.

2 tablespoons ground cinnamon

2 tablespoons paprika

1 tablespoon garlic powder

¼ teaspoon cayenne pepper

4 6-ounce bison filet mignon steaks, cut ¾ to 1 inch thick

2 lemons, halved horizontally

1. In a small bowl stir together the cinnamon, paprika, garlic powder, and cayenne pepper. Pat steaks dry with paper towels. Rub both sides of steaks with the spice mixture.

2. For a charcoal or gas grill, place steaks on the grill rack directly over medium heat. Cover and grill for 10 to 12 minutes for medium rare (145°F) or 12 to 15 minutes for medium (155°F), turning once halfway through grilling. Meanwhile, place lemon halves, cut sides down, on grill rack. Grill for 2 to 3 minutes or until slightly charred and juicy.

3. Serve with grilled lemon halves to squeeze over steaks.

HERBES DE PROVENCE-RUBBED BISON SIRLOIN ROAST

PREP: 15 minutes COOK: 15 minutes ROAST: 1 hour 15 minutes STAND: 15 minutes
MAKES: 4 servings

HERBES DE PROVENCE IS A BLEND OF DRIED HERBS THAT GROW IN PROFUSION IN THE SOUTH OF FRANCE. THE MIX USUALLY CONTAINS SOME COMBINATION OF BASIL, FENNEL SEEDS, LAVENDER, MARJORAM, ROSEMARY, SAGE, SUMMER SAVORY, AND THYME. IT FLAVORS THIS VERY AMERICAN ROAST BEAUTIFULLY.

- 1 3-pound bison sirloin roast
- 3 tablespoons herbes de Provence
- 4 tablespoons extra virgin olive oil
- 3 cloves garlic, minced
- 4 small parsnips, peeled and chopped
- 2 ripe pears, cored and chopped
- ½ cup unsweetened pear nectar
- 1 to 2 teaspoons fresh thyme

1. Preheat oven to 375°F. Trim fat from roast. In a small bowl combine Herbes de Provence, 2 tablespoons of the olive oil, and garlic; rub over the entire roast.

2. Place the roast on a rack in a shallow roasting pan. Insert an oven-going thermometer into the center of the roast.* Roast, uncovered, for 15 minutes. Reduce oven temperature to 300°F. Roast for 60 to 65 minutes more or until meat thermometer registers 140°F (medium rare). Cover with foil and let stand for 15 minutes.

3. Meanwhile, in a large skillet heat the remaining 2 tablespoons olive oil over medium heat. Add parsnips and pears; cook for 10 minutes or until parsnips are crisp-tender, stirring occasionally. Add pear nectar; cook about 5 minutes or until sauce is slightly thickened. Sprinkle with thyme.

4. Thinly slice roast across the grain. Serve meat with parsnips and pears.

*Tip: Bison is very lean and cooks faster than beef. Additionally, the color of the meat is redder than beef, so you can't rely on a visual cue to determine doneness. You will need a meat thermometer to let you know when the meat is done. An oven-going thermometer is ideal, though not a necessity.

COFFEE-BRAISED BISON SHORT RIBS WITH TANGERINE GREMOLATA AND CELERY ROOT MASH

PREP: 15 minutes COOK: 2 hours 45 minutes MAKES: 6 servings

BISON SHORT RIBS ARE BIG AND MEATY. THEY REQUIRE A GOOD LONG COOK IN LIQUID TO GET TENDER. GREMOLATA MADE WITH TANGERINE PEEL BRIGHTENS UP THE FLAVOR OF THIS HEARTY DISH.

MARINADE

    2 cups water

    3 cups strong coffee, chilled

    2 cups fresh tangerine juice

    2 tablespoons snipped fresh rosemary

    1 teaspoon coarsely ground black pepper

    4 pounds bison short ribs, cut between ribs to separate

BRAISE

    2 tablespoons olive oil

    1 teaspoon black pepper

    2 cups chopped onions

    ½ cup chopped shallots

    6 garlic cloves, chopped

    1 jalapeño chile, seeded and chopped (see tip)

    1 cup strong coffee

    1 cup Beef Bone Broth (see recipe) or no-salt-added beef broth

    ¼ cup Paleo Ketchup (see recipe)

    2 tablespoons Dijon-Style Mustard (see recipe)

    3 tablespoons cider vinegar

    Celery Root Mash (see recipe, below)

    Tangerine Gremolata (see recipe, right)

1. For the marinade, in a large nonreactive container (glass or stainless steel) combine water, chilled coffee, tangerine juice, rosemary, and black pepper. Add ribs. Place a plate on top of ribs if necessary to keep them submerged. Cover and chill 4 to 6 hours, rearranging and stirring once.

2. For the braise, preheat oven to 325°F. Drain ribs, discarding marinade. Pat ribs dry with paper towels. In a large Dutch oven heat olive oil over medium-high heat. Season ribs with black pepper. Brown ribs in batches until browned on all sides, about 5 minutes per batch. Transfer to a large plate.

3. Add onions, shallots, garlic, and jalapeño to pot. Reduce heat to medium, cover, and cook until vegetables are soft, stirring occasionally, about 10 minutes. Add coffee and broth; stir, scraping up browned bits. Add Paleo Ketchup, Dijon-Style Mustard, and vinegar. Bring to boiling. Add ribs. Cover and transfer to oven. Cook until meat is tender, about 2 hours 15 minutes, stirring gently and rearranging ribs once or twice.

4. Transfer ribs to a plate; tent with foil to keep warm. Spoon fat from surface of sauce. Boil sauce until reduced to 2 cups, about 5 minutes. Divide Celery Root Mash among 6 plates; top with ribs and sauce. Sprinkle with Tangerine Gremolata.

Celery Root Mash: In a large saucepan combine 3 pounds celery root, peeled and cut into 1-inch pieces and 4 cups Chicken Bone Broth (see recipe) or unsalted chicken broth. Bring to boiling; reduce heat. Drain celery root, reserving broth. Return celery root to saucepan. Add 1 tablespoon olive oil and 2 teaspoons snipped fresh thyme. Using a potato masher, mash the celery root, adding reserved broth, a few tablespoons at a time, as needed to achieve desired consistency.

Tangerine Gremolata: In a small bowl combine ½ cup snipped fresh parsley, 2 tablespoons finely shredded tangerine peel, and 2 cloves minced garlic.

BEEF BONE BROTH

PREP: 25 minutes ROAST: 1 hour COOK: 8 hours MAKES: 8 to 10 cups

BONY OXTAILS MAKE AN EXTREMELY RICH-TASTING BROTH THAT CAN BE USED IN ANY RECIPE THAT CALLS FOR BEEF BROTH—OR SIMPLY ENJOYED AS A PICK-ME-UP IN A MUG ANY TIME OF DAY. THOUGH THEY ACTUALLY USED TO COME FROM AN OX, OXTAILS NOW COME FROM A BEEF ANIMAL.

- 5 carrots, roughly chopped
- 5 stalks celery, roughly chopped
- 2 yellow onions, unpeeled, halved
- 8 ounces white mushrooms
- 1 bulb garlic, unpeeled, halved
- 2 pounds oxtail bones or beef bones
- 2 tomatoes
- 12 cups cold water
- 3 bay leaves

1. Preheat oven to 400°F. In a large rimmed baking sheet or shallow baking pan arrange the carrots, celery, onions, mushrooms, and garlic; place the bones on top of the vegetables. In a food processor pulse tomatoes until smooth. Spread tomatoes over the bones to coat (it's okay if some of the puree drips onto the pan and the vegetables). Roast for 1 to 1½ hours or until bones are deep brown and the vegetables are caramelized. Transfer bones and vegetables to a 10- to 12-quart Dutch oven or stockpot. (If some of the tomato mixture caramelizes on the bottom of the pan, add 1 cup of hot water to the pan and scrape up any bits. Pour the liquid over the bones and

vegetables and reduce water amount by 1 cup.) Add the cold water and bay leaves.

2. Slowly bring the mixture to a simmer over medium-high to high heat. Reduce heat; cover and simmer broth for 8 to 10 hours, stirring occasionally.

3. Strain broth; discard bones and vegetables. Cool broth; transfer broth to storage containers and refrigerate for up to 5 days; freeze for up to 3 months.*

Slow Cooker Directions: For a 6- to 8-quart slow cooker, use 1 pound beef bones, 3 carrots, 3 stalks celery, 1 yellow onion, and 1 bulb garlic. Puree 1 tomato and rub onto the bones. Roast as directed, then transfer the bones and vegetables to the slow cooker. Scrape off any caramelized tomato as directed and add to the slow cooker. Add enough water to cover. Cover and cook on high-heat setting until broth comes to boiling, about 4 hours. Reduce to low-heat setting; cook for 12 to 24 hours. Strain broth; discard bones and vegetables. Store as directed.

*Tip: To easily skim fat off broth, store broth in a covered container in the refrigerator overnight. Fat will rise to the top and form a firm layer that can easily be scraped off. Broth may thicken after chilling.

TUNISIAN SPICE-RUBBED PORK SHOULDER WITH SPICY SWEET POTATO FRIES

PREP: 25 minutes ROAST: 4 hours BAKE: 30 minutes MAKES: 4 servings

THIS IS A GREAT DISH TO MAKE ON A COOL FALL DAY. THE MEAT ROASTS FOR HOURS IN THE OVEN, MAKING YOUR HOUSE SMELL WONDERFUL AND GIVING YOU TIME TO DO OTHER THINGS. OVEN-BAKED SWEET POTATO FRIES DON'T GET CRISP IN THE SAME WAY THAT WHITE POTATOES DO, BUT THEY ARE DELICIOUS IN THEIR OWN WAY, ESPECIALLY WHEN DIPPED IN GARLICKY MAYONNAISE.

PORK
- 1 2½- to 3-pound bone-in pork shoulder roast
- 2 teaspoons ground ancho chile pepper
- 2 teaspoons ground cumin
- 1 teaspoon caraway seeds, lightly crushed
- 1 teaspoon ground coriander
- ½ teaspoon ground turmeric
- ¼ teaspoon ground cinnamon
- 3 tablespoons olive oil

FRIES
- 4 medium sweet potatoes (about 2 pounds), peeled and cut into ½-inch-thick wedges
- ½ teaspoon crushed red pepper
- ½ teaspoon onion powder
- ½ teaspoon garlic powder
- Olive oil
- 1 onion, thinly sliced
- Paleo Aïoli (Garlic Mayo) (see recipe)

1. Preheat oven to 300°F. Trim fat from meat. In a small bowl combine ground ancho chile pepper, ground cumin, caraway seeds, coriander, turmeric, and cinnamon. Sprinkle meat with spice mixture; using your fingers, rub evenly into meat.

2. In an ovenproof 5- to 6-quart Dutch oven heat 1 tablespoon of the olive oil over medium-high heat. Brown pork on all sides in hot oil. Cover and roast about 4 hours or until very tender and meat thermometer registers 190°F. Remove Dutch oven from oven. Let stand, covered, while you prepare the sweet potato fries and the onions, reserving 1 tablespoon of the fat in the Dutch oven.

3. Increase oven temperature to 400°F. For the sweet potato fries, in a large bowl combine sweet potatoes, the remaining 2 tablespoons olive oil, crushed red pepper, onion powder, and garlic powder; toss to coat. Line one large or two small baking sheets with foil; brush with additional olive oil. Arrange sweet potatoes in a single layer on the prepared baking sheet(s). Bake about 30 minutes or until tender, turning the sweet potatoes once halfway through baking.

4. Meanwhile, remove meat from Dutch oven; cover with foil to keep warm. Drain drippings, reserving 1 tablespoon fat. Return the reserved fat to Dutch oven. Add onion; cook over medium heat about 5 minutes or until just softened, stirring occasionally.

5. Transfer the pork and onion to a serving platter. Using two forks, pull the pork into large shreds. Serve pork and fries with Paleo Aïoli.

CUBAN GRILLED PORK SHOULDER

PREP: 15 minutes MARINATE: 24 hours GRILL: 2 hours 30 minutes STAND: 10 minutes
MAKES: 6 to 8 servings

KNOWN AS "LECHON ASADO" IN ITS COUNTRY OF ORIGIN, THIS PORK ROAST IS MARINATED IN A COMBINATION OF FRESH CITRUS JUICES, SPICES, CRUSHED RED PEPPER, AND AN ENTIRE BULB OF MINCED GARLIC. COOKING IT OVER HOT COALS AFTER AN OVERNIGHT SOAK IN THE MARINADE INFUSES IT WITH AMAZING FLAVOR.

- 1 bulb garlic, cloves separated, peeled, and minced
- 1 cup coarsely chopped onions
- 1 cup olive oil
- 1⅓ cups fresh lime juice
- ⅔ cup fresh orange juice
- 1 tablespoon ground cumin
- 1 tablespoon dried oregano, crushed
- 2 teaspoons freshly ground black pepper
- 1 teaspoon crushed red pepper
- 1 4- to 5-pound boneless pork shoulder roast

1. For marinade, separate garlic head into cloves. Peel and mince cloves; place in a large bowl. Add onions, olive oil, lime juice, orange juice, cumin, oregano, black pepper, and crushed red pepper. Stir well and set aside.

2. Using a boning knife, deeply puncture pork roast all over. Carefully lower roast into the marinade, submerging it as much as possible in the liquid. Cover bowl tightly with plastic wrap. Marinate in the refrigerator for 24 hours, turning once.

3. Remove pork from marinade. Pour marinade into a medium saucepan. Bring to boiling; boil for 5 minutes. Remove from heat and let cool. Set aside.

4. For a charcoal grill, arrange medium-hot coals around a drip pan. Test for medium heat above the pan. Place meat on grill rack over drip pan. Cover and grill for 2½ to 3 hours or until an instant-read thermometer inserted into center of roast registers 140°F. (For a gas grill, preheat grill. Reduce heat to medium. Adjust for indirect cooking. Place meat on grill rack over burner that is turned off. Cover and grill as directed.) Remove meat from grill. Cover loosely with foil and let stand for 10 minutes before carving or pulling.

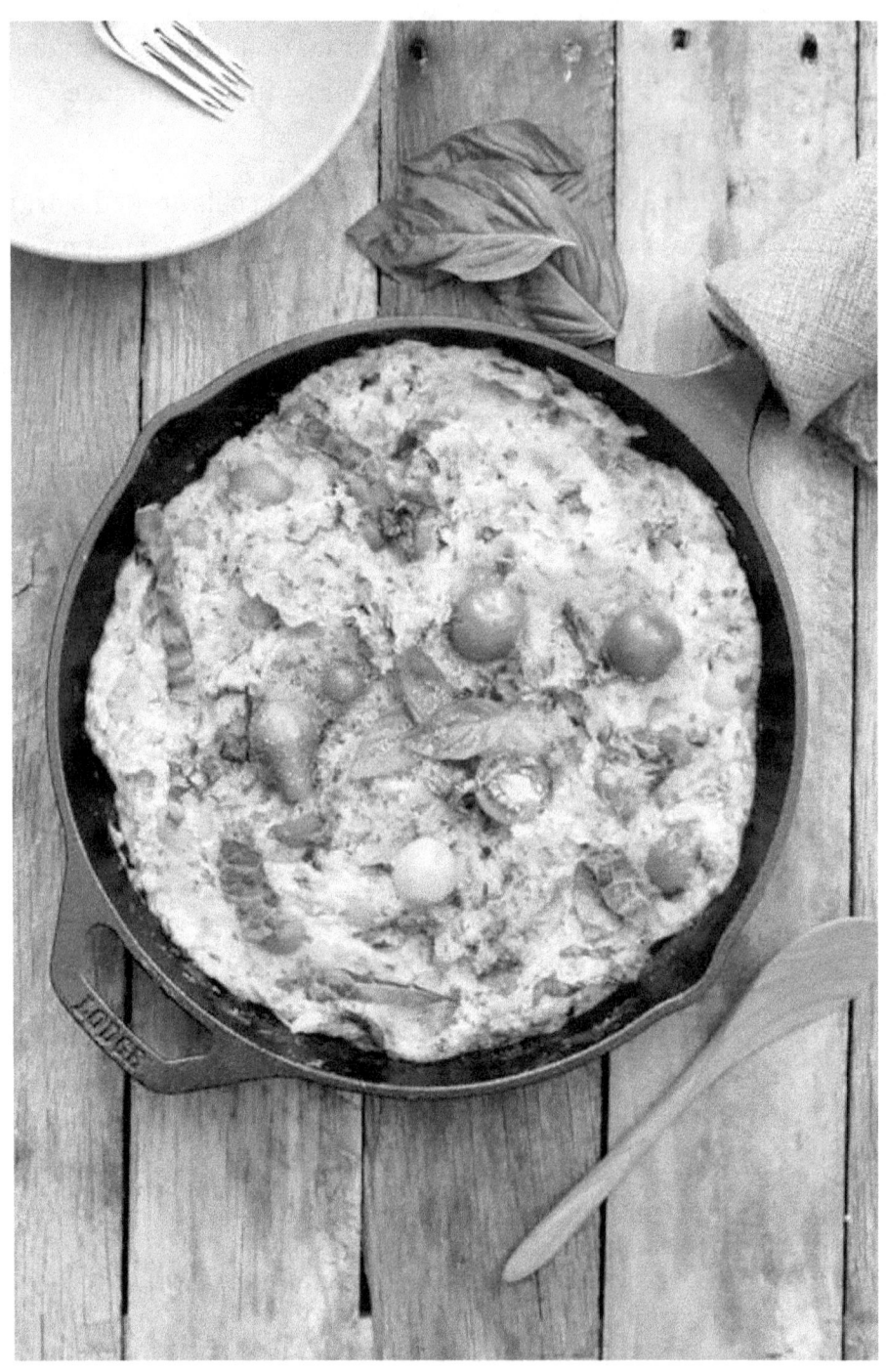

ITALIAN SPICE-RUBBED PORK ROAST WITH VEGETABLES

PREP: 20 minutes ROAST: 2 hours 25 minutes STAND: 10 minutes MAKES: 8 servings

"FRESH IS BEST" IS A GOOD MANTRA TO FOLLOW WHEN IT COMES TO COOKING MOST OF THE TIME. HOWEVER, DRIED HERBS WORK VERY WELL IN RUBS FOR MEATS. WHEN HERBS ARE DRIED, THEIR FLAVORS ARE CONCENTRATED. WHEN THEY COME INTO CONTACT WITH MOISTURE FROM THE MEAT, THEY RELEASE THEIR FLAVORS INTO IT, AS IN THIS ITALIAN-STYLE ROAST FLAVORED WITH PARSLEY, FENNEL, OREGANO, GARLIC, AND SPICY CRUSHED RED PEPPER.

- 2 tablespoons dried parsley, crushed
- 2 tablespoons fennel seeds, crushed
- 4 teaspoons dried oregano, crushed
- 1 teaspoon freshly ground black pepper
- ½ teaspoon crushed red pepper
- 4 cloves garlic, minced
- 1 4-pound bone-in pork shoulder roast
- 1 to 2 tablespoons olive oil
- 1¼ cups water
- 2 medium onions, peeled and cut into wedges
- 1 large fennel bulb, trimmed, cored, and cut into wedges
- 2 pounds Brussels sprouts

1. Preheat oven to 325°F. In a small bowl combine parsley, fennel seeds, oregano, black pepper, crushed red pepper, and garlic; set aside. Untie pork roast if necessary. Trim fat from meat. Rub the meat on all sides with the seasoning mixture. If desired, retie roast to hold it together.

2. In a Dutch oven heat oil over medium-high heat. Brown meat on all sides in the hot oil. Drain off fat. Pour the water into Dutch oven around roast. Roast, uncovered, for 1½ hours. Arrange onions and fennel around pork roast. Cover and roast for 30 minutes more.

3. Meanwhile, trim Brussels sprouts stems and remove any wilted outer leaves. Cut Brussels sprouts in half. Add Brussels sprouts to Dutch oven, arranging them over other vegetables. Cover and roast for 30 to 35 minutes more or until vegetables and meat are tender. Transfer meat to a serving platter and cover with foil. Let stand for 15 minutes before slicing. Toss vegetables with pan juices to coat. Using a slotted spoon, remove vegetables to the serving platter or a bowl; cover to keep warm.

4. Using a large spoon, skim fat from pan juices. Pour remaining pan juices through a sieve. Slice pork, removing the bone. Serve meat with vegetables and pan juices.

SLOW COOKER PORK MOLE

PREP: 20 minutes SLOW COOK: 8 to 10 hours (low) or 4 to 5 hours (high) MAKES: 8 servings

WITH CUMIN, CORIANDER, OREGANO, TOMATOES, ALMONDS, RAISINS, CHILE, AND CHOCOLATE, THIS RICH AND SPICY SAUCE HAS A LOT GOING ON—IN A VERY GOOD WAY. IT'S AN IDEAL MEAL TO START IN THE MORNING BEFORE YOU HEAD OUT FOR THE DAY. WHEN YOU COME HOME, DINNER IS NEARLY DONE—AND YOUR HOUSE SMELLS AMAZING.

- 1 3-pound boneless pork shoulder roast
- 1 cup coarsely chopped onion
- 3 cloves garlic, sliced
- 1½ cups Beef Bone Broth (see recipe), Chicken Bone Broth (see recipe), or no-salt-added beef or chicken broth
- 1 tablespoon ground cumin
- 1 tablespoon ground coriander
- 2 teaspoons dried oregano, crushed
- 1 15-ounce can diced no-salt-added tomatoes, drained
- 1 6-ounce can no-salt-added tomato paste
- ½ cup slivered almonds, toasted (see tip)
- ¼ cup unsulfured golden raisins or currants
- 2 ounces unsweetened chocolate (such as Scharffen Berger 99% cacao bar), coarsely chopped
- 1 dried whole ancho or chipotle chile pepper
- 2 4-inch cinnamon sticks
- ¼ cup snipped fresh cilantro
- 1 avocado, peeled, seeded, and thinly sliced
- 1 lime, cut into wedges
- ⅓ cup toasted unsalted green pumpkin seeds (optional) (see tip)

1. Trim fat from pork roast. If necessary, cut meat to fit a 5- to 6-quart slow cooker; set aside.

2. In the slow cooker combine onion and garlic. In a 2-cup glass measuring cup stir together Beef Bone Broth, cumin, coriander, and oregano; pour into cooker. Stir in diced tomatoes, tomato paste, almonds, raisins, chocolate, dried chile pepper, and cinnamon sticks. Place meat in cooker. Spoon some of the tomato mixture over the top. Cover and cook on low-heat setting for 8 to 10 hours or on high-heat setting for 4 to 5 hours or until pork is tender.

3. Transfer pork to a cutting board; cool slightly. Using two forks, pull meat apart into shreds. Cover meat with foil and set aside.

4. Remove and discard dried chile pepper and cinnamon sticks. Using a large spoon, skim fat from tomato mixture. Transfer the tomato mixture to a blender or food processor. Cover and blend or process until almost smooth. Return pulled pork and sauce into slow cooker. Keep warm on low-heat setting until serving time, up to 2 hours.

5. Just before serving, stir in cilantro. Serve mole in bowls and garnish with avocado slices, lime wedges, and, if desired, pumpkin seeds.

CARAWAY-SPICED PORK AND SQUASH STEW

PREP: 30 minutes COOK: 1 hour MAKES: 4 servings

PEPPERY MUSTARD GREENS AND BUTTERNUT SQUASH ADD VIBRANT COLOR AND A WHOLE HOST OF VITAMINS—AS WELL AS FIBER AND FOLIC ACID—TO THIS STEW SPICED WITH EASTERN EUROPEAN FLAVORS.

- 1 1¼- to 1½-pound pork shoulder roast
- 1 tablespoon paprika
- 1 tablespoon caraway seeds, finely crushed
- 2 teaspoons dry mustard
- ¼ teaspoon cayenne pepper
- 2 tablespoon refined coconut oil
- 8 ounces fresh button mushrooms, thinly sliced
- 2 stalks celery, cut crosswise into 1-inch slices
- 1 small red onion, cut into thin wedges
- 6 cloves garlic, minced
- 5 cups Chicken Bone Broth (see <u>recipe</u>) or no-salt-added chicken broth
- 2 cups cubed, peeled butternut squash
- 3 cups coarsely chopped, trimmed mustard greens or green cabbage
- 2 tablespoons snipped fresh sage
- ¼ cup fresh lemon juice

1. Trim fat from pork. Cut pork into 1½-inch cubes; place in a large bowl. In a small bowl combine paprika, caraway seeds, dry mustard, and cayenne pepper. Sprinkle over pork, tossing to coat evenly.

2. In a 4- to 5-quart Dutch oven heat coconut oil over medium heat. Add half of the meat; cook until browned, stirring

occasionally. Remove meat from the pan. Repeat with the remaining meat. Set meat aside.

3. Add mushrooms, celery, red onion, and garlic to Dutch oven. Cook for 5 minutes, stirring occasionally. Return meat to the Dutch oven. Carefully add Chicken Bone Broth. Bring to boiling; reduce heat. Cover and simmer for 45 minutes. Stir in squash. Cover and simmer for 10 to 15 minutes more or until pork and squash are tender. Stir in mustard greens and sage. Cook for 2 to 3 minutes or until greens are just tender. Stir in lemon juice.

FRUIT-STUFFED TOP LOIN ROAST WITH BRANDY SAUCE

PREP: 30 minutes COOK: 10 minutes ROAST: 1 hour 15 minutes STAND: 15 minutes
MAKES: 8 to 10 servings

THIS ELEGANT ROAST IS PERFECT FOR A SPECIAL OCCASION OR FAMILY GATHERING—PARTICULARLY IN THE FALL. ITS FLAVORS—APPLES, NUTMEG, DRIED FRUIT, AND PECANS—CAPTURE THE ESSENCE OF THAT SEASON. SERVE IT WITH MASHED SWEET POTATOES AND BLUEBERRY AND ROASTED BEET KALE SALAD (SEE RECIPE).

ROAST
- 1 tablespoon olive oil
- 2 cups chopped, peeled Granny Smith apples (about 2 medium)
- 1 shallot, finely chopped
- 1 tablespoon snipped fresh thyme
- ¾ teaspoon freshly ground black pepper
- ⅛ teaspoon ground nutmeg
- ½ cup snipped unsulfured dried apricots
- ¼ cup chopped pecans, toasted (see tip)
- 1 cup Chicken Bone Broth (see recipe) or no-salt-added chicken broth
- 1 3-pound boneless pork top loin roast (single loin)

BRANDY SAUCE
- 2 tablespoons apple cider
- 2 tablespoons brandy
- 1 teaspoon Dijon-Style Mustard (see recipe)
- Freshly ground black pepper

1. For the stuffing, in a large skillet heat olive oil over medium heat. Add apples, shallot, thyme, ¼ teaspoon of the pepper, and nutmeg; cook for 2 to 4 minutes or until

apples and shallot are tender and light golden, stirring occasionally. Stir in apricots, pecans, and 1 tablespoon of the broth. Cook, uncovered, for 1 minute to soften apricots. Remove from heat and set aside.

2. Preheat oven to 325°F. Butterfly the pork roast by making a lengthwise cut down the center of the roast, cutting to within ½ inch of the other side. Spread the roast open. Place the knife in the V cut, facing it horizontally toward one side of the V, and cut to within ½ inch of the side. Repeat on the other side of the V. Spread the roast open and cover with plastic wrap. Working from the center to the edges, pound the roast with a meat mallet until it is about ¾ inch thick. Remove and discard plastic wrap. Spread the stuffing over the top of the roast. Starting from a short side, roll the roast into a spiral. Tie with 100%-cotton kitchen string in several places to hold the roast together. Sprinkle roast with the remaining ½ teaspoon pepper.

3. Place roast on a rack in a shallow roasting pan. Insert an oven-going thermometer into the center of the roast (not in the stuffing). Roast, uncovered, for 1 hour 15 minutes to 1 hour 30 minutes or until thermometer registers 145°F. Remove roast and cover loosely with foil; let stand for 15 minutes before slicing.

4. Meanwhile, for Brandy Sauce, stir the remaining broth and apple cider into drippings in pan, whisking to scrape up browned bits. Strain drippings into a medium saucepan. Bring to boiling; cook about 4 minutes or until sauce is reduced by one-third. Stir in brandy and Dijon-Style

Mustard. Season to taste with additional pepper. Serve sauce with the pork roast.

PORCHETTA-STYLE PORK ROAST

PREP: 15 minutes MARINATE: overnight STAND: 40 minutes ROAST: 1 hour MAKES: 6 servings

TRADITIONAL ITALIAN PORCHETTA (SOMETIMES SPELLED PORKETTA IN AMERICAN ENGLISH) IS A BONELESS SUCKLING PIG STUFFED WITH GARLIC, FENNEL, PEPPER, AND HERBS SUCH AS SAGE OR ROSEMARY, THEN PUT ON A SPIT AND ROASTED OVER WOOD. IT'S ALSO USUALLY HEAVILY SALTED. THIS PALEO VERSION IS SIMPLIFIED AND VERY TASTY. SUBSTITUTE FRESH ROSEMARY FOR THE SAGE, IF YOU LIKE, OR USE A BLEND OF THE TWO HERBS.

- 1 2- to 3-pound boneless pork loin roast
- 2 tablespoons fennel seeds
- 1 teaspoon black peppercorns
- ½ teaspoon crushed red pepper
- 6 cloves garlic, minced
- 1 tablespoon finely shredded orange peel
- 1 tablespoon snipped fresh sage
- 3 tablespoon olive oil
- ½ cup dry white wine
- ½ cup Chicken Bone Broth (see recipe) or no-salt-added chicken broth

1. Remove pork roast from refrigerator; let stand at room temperature for 30 minutes. Meanwhile, in a small skillet toast fennel seeds over medium heat, stirring frequently, about 3 minutes or until dark in color and fragrant; cool. Transfer to a spice mill or clean coffee grinder. Add peppercorns and crushed red pepper. Grind to medium-fine consistency. (Do not grind to a powder.)

2. Preheat oven to 325°F. In a small bowl combine ground spices, garlic, orange peel, sage, and olive oil to make a paste. Place pork roast on a rack in a small roasting pan. Rub mixture all over pork. (If desired, place seasoned pork in a 9×13×2-inch glass baking dish. Cover with with plastic wrap and refrigerate overnight to marinate. Transfer meat to a roasting pan before cooking and let stand at room temperature for 30 minutes before cooking.)

3. Roast pork for 1 to 1½ hours or until an instant-read thermometer inserted into center of roast registers 145°F. Transfer roast to a cutting board and cover loosely with foil. Let stand for 10 to 15 minutes before slicing.

4. Meanwhile, pour pan juices into a glass measuring cup. Skim fat from top; set aside. Place roasting pan on stovetop burner. Pour wine and Chicken Bone Broth into pan. Bring to boiling over medium-high heat, stirring to scrape up any browned bits. Boil about 4 minutes or until mixture is slightly reduced. Whisk in reserved pan juices; strain. Slice pork and serve with sauce.

TOMATILLO-BRAISED PORK LOIN

PREP: 40 minutes BROIL: 10 minutes COOK: 20 minutes ROAST: 40 minutes STAND: 10 minutes MAKES: 6 to 8 servings

TOMATILLOS HAVE A STICKY, SAPPY COATING UNDER THEIR PAPER SKINS. AFTER YOU REMOVE THE SKINS, GIVE THEM A QUICK RINSE UNDER RUNNING WATER AND THEY ARE READY TO USE.

1 pound tomatillos, husked, stemmed, and rinsed
4 serrano chiles, stemmed, seeded, and halved (see tip)
2 jalapeños, stemmed, seeded, and halved (see tip)
1 large yellow sweet pepper, stemmed, seeded, and halved
1 large orange sweet pepper, stemmed, seeded, and halved
2 tablespoons olive oil
1 2- to 2½-pound boneless pork loin roast
1 large yellow onion, peeled, halved, and thinly sliced
4 cloves garlic, minced
¾ cup water
¼ cup fresh lime juice
¼ cup snipped fresh cilantro

1. Preheat broiler to high. Line a baking sheet with foil. Arrange tomatillos, serrano chiles, jalapeños, and sweet peppers on prepared baking sheet. Broil vegetables 4 inches from heat until well charred, turning tomatillos occasionally and removing vegetables as they become charred, about 10 to 15 minutes. Place serranos, jalapeños, and tomatillos in a bowl. Place sweet peppers on a plate. Set vegetables aside to cool.

2. In a large skillet heat oil over medium-high heat until it shimmers. Pat pork roast dry with clean paper towels and add to skillet. Cook until well browned on all sides,

turning roast to brown evenly. Transfer roast to a platter. Reduce heat to medium. Add onion to skillet; cook and stir for 5 to 6 minutes or until golden. Add garlic; cook for 1 minute more. Remove skillet from heat.

3. Preheat oven to 350°F. For tomatillo sauce, in a food processor or blender combine tomatillos, serranos, and jalapeños. Cover and blend or process until smooth; add to onion in skillet. Return skillet to heat. Bring to boiling; cook for 4 to 5 minutes or until mixture is dark and thick. Stir in the water, lime juice, and cilantro.

4. Spread tomatillo sauce in a shallow roasting pan or 3-quart rectangular baking dish. Place pork roast in the sauce. Cover tightly with foil. Roast for 40 to 45 minutes or until an instant-read thermometer inserted into the center of the roast reads 140°F.

5. Cut sweet peppers into strips. Stir into the tomatillo sauce in pan. Tent loosely with foil; let stand for 10 minutes. Slice meat; stir sauce. Serve sliced pork topped generously with tomatillo sauce.

APRICOT-STUFFED PORK TENDERLOIN

PREP: 20 minutes ROAST: 45 minutes STAND: 5 minutes MAKES: 2 to 3 servings

- 2 medium fresh apricots, coarsely chopped
- 2 tablespoons unsulfured raisins
- 2 tablespoons chopped walnuts
- 2 teaspoons grated fresh ginger
- ¼ teaspoon ground cardamom
- 1 12-ounce pork tenderloin
- 1 tablespoon olive oil
- 1 tablespoon Dijon-Style Mustard (see recipe)
- ¼ teaspoon black pepper

1. Preheat oven to 375°F. Line a baking sheet with foil; place a roasting rack on the baking sheet.

2. In a small bowl stir together the apricots, raisins, walnuts, ginger, and cardamom.

3. Make a lengthwise cut down the center of the pork, cutting to within ½ inch of the other side. Butterfly it open. Place the pork between two layers of plastic wrap. Using the flat side of a meat mallet, lightly pound meat until about ⅓ inch thick. Fold in the tail end to make an even rectangle. Lightly pound meat to make even thickness.

4. Spread the apricot mixture over the pork. Beginning at the narrow end, roll up the pork. Tie with 100%-cotton kitchen string, first in the center, then at 1-inch intervals. Place roast on the rack.

5. Stir together the olive oil and Dijon-Style Mustard; brush over the roast. Sprinkle roast with pepper. Roast for 45 to

55 minutes or until an instant-read thermometer inserted into center of roast registers 140°F. Let stand for 5 to 10 minutes before slicing.

HERB-CRUSTED PORK TENDERLOIN WITH CRISPY GARLIC OIL

PREP: 15 minutes ROAST: 30 minutes COOK: 8 minutes STAND: 5 minutes MAKES: 6 servings

⅓ cup Dijon-Style Mustard (see recipe)
¼ cup snipped fresh parsley
2 tablespoons snipped fresh thyme
1 tablespoon snipped fresh rosemary
½ teaspoon black pepper
2 12-ounce pork tenderloins
½ cup olive oil
¼ cup minced fresh garlic
¼ to 1 teaspoon crushed red pepper

1. Preheat oven to 450°F. Line a baking sheet with foil; place a roasting rack on the baking sheet.

2. In a small bowl stir together the mustard, parsley, thyme, rosemary, and black pepper to make a paste. Spread the mustard-herb mixture over the top and sides of the pork. Transfer pork to the roasting rack. Place roast in the oven; decrease temperature to 375°F. Roast for 30 to 35 minutes or until an instant-read thermometer inserted into center of roast registers 140°F. Let stand for 5 to 10 minutes before slicing.

3. Meanwhile, for garlic oil, in a small saucepan combine the olive oil and garlic. Cook over medium-low heat for 8 to 10 minutes or until garlic is golden and begins to crisp (do not let garlic burn). Remove from heat; stir in crushed red pepper. Slice pork; spoon garlic oil over the slices before serving.

INDIAN-SPICED PORK WITH COCONUT PAN SAUCE

START TO FINISH: 20 minutes MAKES: 2 servings

3 teaspoons curry powder
2 teaspoons salt-free garam masala
1 teaspoon ground cumin
1 teaspoon ground coriander
1 12-ounce pork tenderloin
1 tablespoon olive oil
½ cup natural coconut milk (such as Nature's Way brand)
¼ cup snipped fresh cilantro
2 tablespoons snipped fresh mint

1. In a small bowl stir together 2 teaspoons of the curry powder, garam masala, cumin, and coriander. Slice pork into ½-inch-thick slices; sprinkle with spices. .

2. In a large skillet heat olive oil over medium heat. Add pork slices to skillet; cook for 7 minutes, turning once. Remove pork from skillet; cover to keep warm. For sauce, add coconut milk and the remaining 1 teaspoon curry powder to the skillet, stirring to scrape up any bits. Simmer for 2 to 3 minutes. Stir in cilantro and mint. Add pork; cook until heated through, spooning sauce over the pork.

PORK SCALOPPINI WITH SPICED APPLES AND CHESTNUTS

PREP: 20 minutes COOK: 15 minutes MAKES: 4 servings

2 12-ounce pork tenderloins
1 tablespoon onion powder
1 tablespoon garlic powder
½ teaspoon black pepper
2 to 4 tablespoons olive oil
2 Fuji or Pink Lady apples, peeled, cored, and coarsely chopped
¼ cup finely chopped shallots
¾ teaspoon ground cinnamon
⅛ teaspoon ground cloves
⅛ teaspoon ground nutmeg
½ cup Chicken Bone Broth (see <u>recipe</u>) or no-salt added chicken broth
2 tablespoons fresh lemon juice
½ cup peeled roasted chestnuts, chopped,* or chopped pecans
1 tablespoon snipped fresh sage

1. Cut the tenderloins into ½-inch- thick slices on a bias. Place pork slices between two sheets of plastic wrap. Using the flat side of a meat mallet, pound until thin. Sprinkle slices with onion powder, garlic powder, and black pepper.

2. In a large skillet heat 2 tablespoons olive oil over medium heat. Cook pork, in batches, for 3 to 4 minutes, turning once and adding oil if necessary. Transfer pork to a plate; cover and keep warm.

3. Increase heat to medium-high. Add the apples, shallots, cinnamon, cloves, and nutmeg. Cook and stir for 3 minutes. Stir in Chicken Bone Broth and lemon juice.

Cover and cook for 5 minutes. Remove from heat; stir in the chestnuts and sage. Serve apple mixture over pork.

*Note: To roast chestnuts, preheat oven to 400°F. Cut an X in one side of the chestnut shell. This will let the shell loosen as it cooks. Place chestnuts on a baking pan and roast for 30 minutes or until the shell pulls apart from the nut and the nuts are tender. Wrap the roasted chestnuts in a clean kitchen towel. Peel shells and skin from the yellow-white nut.

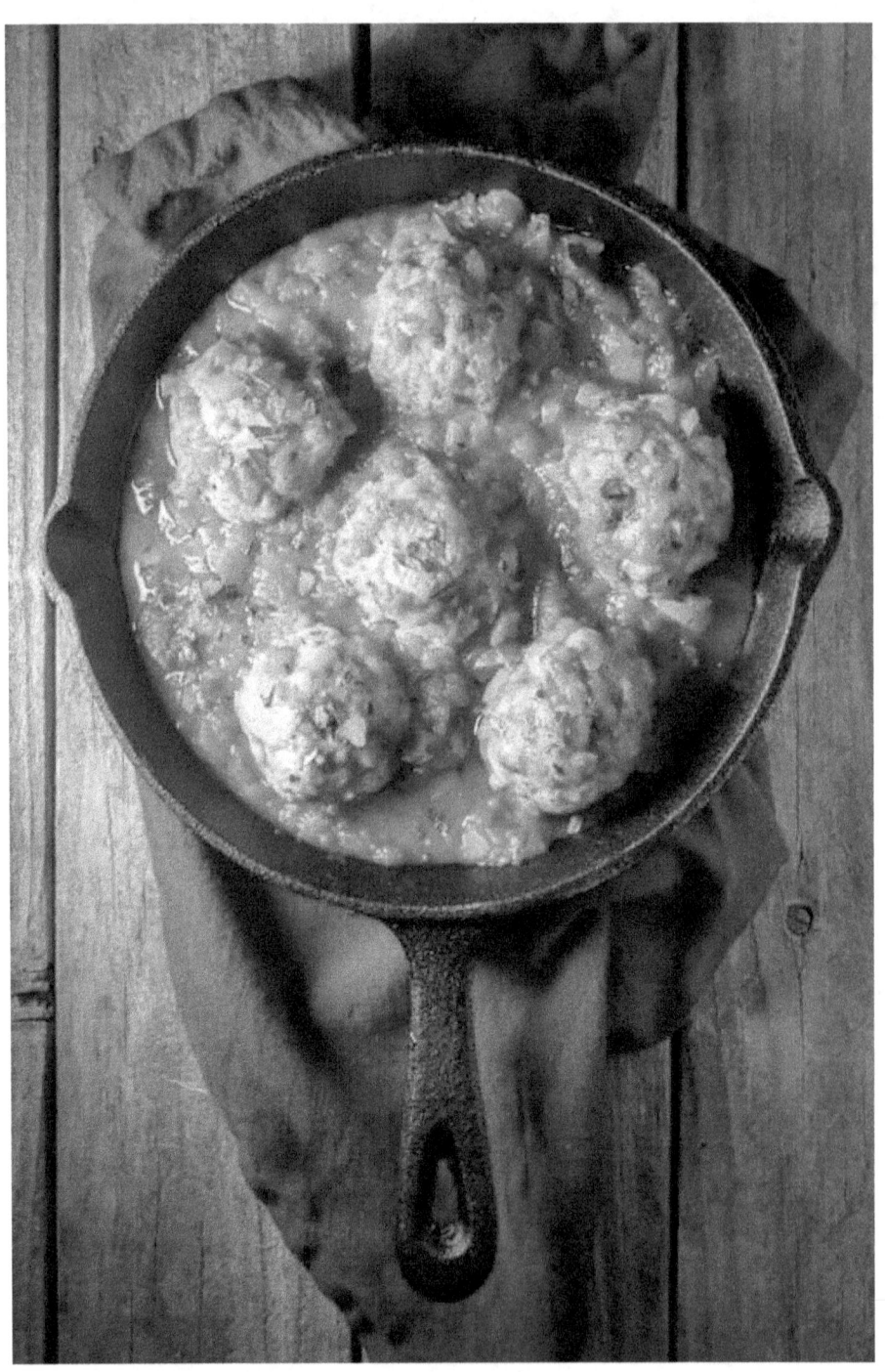

PORK FAJITA STIR-FRY

PREP: 20 minutes COOK: 22 minutes MAKES: 4 servings

- 1 pound pork tenderloin, cut into 2-inch strips
- 3 tablespoons salt-free fajita seasoning or Mexican Seasoning (see recipe)
- 2 tablespoons olive oil
- 1 small onion, thinly sliced
- ½ of a red sweet pepper, seeded and thinly sliced
- ½ of an orange sweet pepper, seeded and thinly sliced
- 1 jalapeño, stemmed and thinly sliced (see tip) (optional)
- ½ teaspoon cumin seeds
- 1 cup thinly sliced fresh mushrooms
- 3 tablespoons fresh lime juice
- ½ cup snipped fresh cilantro
- 1 avocado, seeded, peeled, and diced
- Desired salsa (see recipes)

1. Sprinkle the pork with 2 tablespoons fajita seasoning. In an extra-large skillet heat 1 tablespoon of the oil over medium-high heat. Add half the pork; cook and stir about 5 minutes or until no longer pink. Transfer meat to a bowl and cover to keep warm. Repeat with remaining oil and pork.

2. Turn heat to medium. Add the remaining 1 tablespoon fajita seasoning, onion, sweet peppers, jalapeño, and cumin. Cook and stir about 10 minutes or until vegetables are tender. Return all the meat and accumulated juices to skillet. Stir in mushrooms and lime juice. Cook until heated through. Remove skillet from heat; stir in the cilantro. Serve with avocado and desired salsa.

PORK TENDERLOIN WITH PORT AND PRUNES

PREP: 10 minutes ROAST: 12 minutes STAND: 5 minutes MAKES: 4 servings

PORT IS A FORTIFIED WINE, WHICH MEANS IT HAS A SPIRIT SIMILAR TO BRANDY ADDED TO IT TO STOP THE FERMENTATION PROCESS. THIS MEANS THERE IS MORE RESIDUAL SUGAR IN IT THAN RED TABLE WINE AND CONSEQUENTLY IT HAS A SWEETER TASTE. IT ISN'T SOMETHING YOU WANT TO DRINK EVERY DAY, BUT A LITTLE BIT USED IN COOKING ONCE IN A WHILE IS FINE.

- 2 12-ounce pork tenderloins
- 2½ teaspoons ground coriander
- ¼ teaspoon black pepper
- 2 tablespoons olive oil
- 1 shallot, sliced
- ½ cup port wine
- ½ cup Chicken Bone Broth (see recipe) or no-salt-added chicken broth
- 20 pitted unsulfured dried plums (prunes)
- ½ teaspoon crushed red pepper
- 2 teaspoons snipped fresh tarragon

1. Preheat oven to 400°F. Sprinkle pork with 2 teaspoons of the coriander and the black pepper.

2. In a large ovenproof skillet heat olive oil over medium-high heat. Add tenderloins to skillet. Cook until browned on all sides, turning to brown evenly, about 8 minutes. Place skillet in oven. Roast, uncovered, about 12 minutes or until an instant-read thermometer inserted into center of roasts registers 140°F. Transfer tenderloins to a cutting

board. Cover loosely with aluminum foil and let stand for 5 minutes.

3. Meanwhile, for sauce, drain fat from skillet, reserving 1 tablespoon. Cook shallot in the reserved drippings in skillet over medium heat about 3 minutes or until browned and tender. Add port to skillet. Bring to boiling, stirring to scrape up any browned bits. Add Chicken Bone Broth, dried plums, crushed red pepper, and the remaining ½ teaspoon coriander. Cook over medium-high heat to reduce slightly, about 1 to 2 minutes. Stir in tarragon.

4. Slice pork and serve with prunes and sauce.

MOO SHU-STYLE PORK IN LETTUCE CUPS WITH QUICK PICKLED VEGETABLES

START TO FINISH: 45 minutes MAKES: 4 servings

IF YOU'VE HAD A TRADITIONAL MOO SHU DISH IN A CHINESE RESTAURANT, YOU KNOW IT IS A SAVORY MEAT AND VEGETABLE FILLING EATEN IN THIN PANCAKES WITH A SWEET PLUM OR HOISIN SAUCE. THIS LIGHTER AND FRESHER PALEO VERSION FEATURES PORK, CHINESE CABBAGE, AND SHIITAKE MUSHROOMS STIR-FRIED IN GINGER AND GARLIC AND ENJOYED IN LETTUCE WRAPS WITH CRUNCHY PICKLED VEGETABLES.

PICKLED VEGETABLES

- 1 cup julienne-cut carrots
- 1 cup julienne-cut daikon radish
- ¼ cup slivered red onion
- 1 cup unsweetened apple juice
- ½ cup cider vinegar

PORK

- 2 tablespoons olive oil or refined coconut oil
- 3 eggs, lightly beaten
- 8 ounces pork loin, cut into 2×½-inch strips
- 2 teaspoons minced fresh ginger
- 4 cloves garlic, minced
- 2 cups thinly sliced napa cabbage
- 1 cup thinly sliced shiitake mushrooms
- ¼ cup thinly sliced scallions
- 8 Boston lettuce leaves

1. For quick pickled vegetables, in a large bowl toss together the carrots, daikon, and onion. For brine, in a saucepan heat the apple juice and vinegar just until steam rises. Pour the brine over the vegetables in bowl; cover and chill until ready to serve.

2. In a large skillet heat 1 tablespoon of the oil over medium-high heat. Using a whisk, lightly beat eggs. Add eggs to skillet; cook, without stirring, until set on the bottom, about 3 minutes. Using a flexible spatula, carefully turn the egg over and cook on the other side. Slide the egg out of the pan onto a platter.

3. Return the skillet to heat; add the remaining 1 tablespoon oil. Add the pork strips, ginger, and garlic. Cook and stir over medium-high heat about 4 minutes or until pork is no longer pink. Add the cabbage and mushrooms; cook and stir about 4 minutes or until cabbage wilts, mushrooms soften, and pork is cooked through. Remove skillet from heat. Cut the cooked egg into strips. Gently stir egg strips and scallions into pork mixture. Serve in lettuce leaves and top with pickled vegetables.

PORK CHOPS WITH MACADAMIAS, SAGE, FIGS, AND MASHED SWEET POTATOES

PREP: 15 minutes COOK: 25 minutes MAKES: 4 servings

PAIRED WITH MASHED SWEET POTATOES, THESE JUICY SAGE-TOPPED CHOPS MAKE A PERFECT FALL MEAL—AND ONE THAT'S QUICK TO FIX, MAKING IT A PERFECT FOR A BUSY WEEKNIGHT.

4 boneless pork loin chops, cut 1¼ inches thick
3 tablespoons snipped fresh sage
¼ teaspoon black pepper
3 tablespoons macadamia nut oil
2 pounds sweet potatoes, peeled and cut into 1-inch pieces
¾ cup chopped macadamia nuts
½ cup chopped dried figs
⅓ cup Beef Bone Broth (see recipe) or no-salt-added beef broth
1 tablespoon fresh lemon juice

1. Sprinkle both sides of pork chops with 2 tablespoons of the sage and the pepper; rub in with your fingers. In a large skillet heat 2 tablespoons of the oil over medium heat. Add chops to skillet; cook for 15 to 20 minutes or until done (145°F), turning once halfway through cooking. Transfer chops to a plate; cover to keep warm.

2. Meanwhile, in a large saucepan combine sweet potatoes and enough water to cover. Bring to boiling; reduce heat. Cover and simmer for 10 to 15 minutes or until potatoes are tender. Drain potatoes. Add the remaining tablespoon macadamia oil to potatoes and mash until creamy; keep warm.

3. For sauce, add macadamia nuts to skillet; cook over medium heat just until toasted. Add dried figs and the remaining 1 tablespoon sage; cook for 30 seconds. Add Beef Bone Broth and lemon juice to skillet, stirring to scrape up any browned bits. Spoon sauce over pork chops and serve with mashed sweet potatoes.

SKILLET-ROASTED ROSEMARY-LAVENDER PORK CHOPS WITH GRAPES AND TOASTED WALNUTS

PREP: 10 minutes COOK: 6 minutes ROAST: 25 minutes MAKES: 4 servings

ROASTING THE GRAPES ALONG WITH THE PORK CHOPS INTENSIFIES THEIR FLAVOR AND SWEETNESS. ALONG WITH THE CRUNCHY TOASTED WALNUTS AND A SPRINKLING OF FRESH ROSEMARY, THEY MAKE A WONDERFUL TOPPING FOR THESE HEARTY CHOPS.

2 tablespoons snipped fresh rosemary

1 tablespoon snipped fresh lavender

½ teaspoon garlic powder

½ teaspoon black pepper

4 pork loin chops, cut 1¼ inches thick (about 3 pounds)

1 tablespoon olive oil

1 large shallot, thinly sliced

1½ cups red and/or green seedless grapes

½ cup dry white wine

¾ cup coarsely chopped walnuts

Snipped fresh rosemary

1. Preheat oven to 375°F. In a small bowl combine 2 tablespoons rosemary, lavender, garlic powder, and pepper. Rub herb mixture evenly into pork chops. In an extra-large ovenproof skillet heat olive oil over medium heat. Add chops to skillet; cook for 6 to 8 minutes or until browned on both sides. Transfer chops to a plate; cover with foil.

2. Add the shallot to the skillet. Cook and stir over medium heat for 1 minute. Add grapes and wine. Cook about 2 minutes more, stirring to scrape up any browned bits. Return pork chops to skillet. Place the skillet in the oven; roast for 25 to 30 minutes or until chops are done (145°F).

3. Meanwhile, spread the walnuts in a shallow baking pan. Add to oven with chops. Roast about 8 minutes or until toasted, stirring once to toast evenly.

4. To serve, top pork chops with grapes and toasted walnuts. Sprinkle with additional fresh rosemary.

PORK CHOPS ALLA FIORENTINA WITH GRILLED BROCCOLI RABE

PREP: 20 minutes GRILL: 20 minutes MARINATE: 3 minutes MAKES: 4 servings PHOTO

"ALLA FIORENTINA" ESSENTIALLY MEANS "IN THE STYLE OF FLORENCE." THIS RECIPE IS STYLED AFTER *BISTECCA ALLA FIORENTINA*, A TUSCAN T-BONE GRILLED OVER A WOOD FIRE WITH THE SIMPLEST FLAVORINGS—USUALLY JUST OLIVE OIL, SALT, BLACK PEPPER, AND A SQUEEZE OF FRESH LEMON TO FINISH.

1 pound broccoli rabe
1 tablespoon olive oil
4 6- to 8-ounce bone-in pork loin chops, cut 1½ to 2 inches thick
Coarsely ground black pepper
1 lemon
4 cloves garlic, thinly sliced
2 tablespoons snipped fresh rosemary
6 fresh sage leaves, chopped
1 teaspoon crushed red pepper flakes (or to taste)
½ cup olive oil

1. In a large saucepan blanch the broccoli rabe in boiling water for 1 minute. Immediately transfer to a bowl of ice water. When cool, drain the broccoli rabe on a paper towel-lined baking sheet, blotting as dry as possible with additional paper towels. Remove paper towels from baking sheet. Drizzle the broccoli rabe with 1 tablespoon olive oil, tossing to coat; set aside until ready to grill.

2. Sprinkle both sides of the pork chops with coarsely ground pepper; set aside. Using a vegetable peeler, remove strips

of peel from lemon (save lemon for another use). Scatter lemon peel strips, sliced garlic, rosemary, sage, and crushed red pepper on a large serving platter; set aside.

3. For a charcoal grill, move most hot coals to one side of the grill, leaving some coals under the other side of the grill. Sear the chops directly over the hot coals for 2 to 3 minutes or until a brown crust forms. Turn the chops over and sear on the second side for 2 minutes more. Move the chops to the other side of the grill. Cover and grill for 10 to 15 minutes or until done (145°F). (For a gas grill, preheat grill; reduce heat on one side of grill to medium. Sear chops as directed above over high heat. Move to medium heat side of grill; continue as directed above.)

4. Transfer the chops to the platter. Drizzle chops with the ½ cup olive oil, turning to coat both sides. Let the chops marinate for 3 to 5 minutes before serving, turning once or twice to infuse the meat with the flavors of the lemon peel, garlic, and herbs.

5. While the chops rest, grill the broccoli rabe to char lightly and warm through. Arrange broccoli rabe on the platter with the pork chops; spoon some of the marinade over each chop and broccoli rabe before serving.

ESCAROLE-STUFFED PORK CHOPS

PREP: 20 minutes COOK: 9 minutes MAKES: 4 servings

ESCAROLE CAN BE EATEN AS A SALAD GREEN OR LIGHTLY SAUTÉED WITH GARLIC IN OLIVE OIL FOR A QUICK SIDE DISH. HERE, COMBINED WITH OLIVE OIL, GARLIC, BLACK PEPPER, CRUSHED RED PEPPER, AND LEMON, IT MAKES A BEAUTIFUL BRIGHT-GREEN FILLING FOR JUICY PAN-SEARED PORK CHOPS.

4 6- to 8-ounce bone-in pork chops, cut ¾ inch thick
½ of a medium head escarole, finely chopped
4 tablespoons olive oil
1 tablespoon fresh lemon juice
¼ teaspoon black pepper
¼ teaspoon crushed red pepper
2 large cloves garlic, minced
Olive oil
1 tablespoon snipped fresh sage
¼ teaspoon black pepper
⅓ cup dry white wine

1. Using a paring knife, cut a deep pocket, about 2 inches wide, into the curved side of each pork chop; set aside.

2. In a large bowl combine escarole, 2 tablespoons of the olive oil, lemon juice, ¼ teaspoon black pepper, crushed red pepper, and garlic. Stuff each chop with one-fourth of the mixture. Brush chops with olive oil. Sprinkle with sage and ¼ teaspoon ground black pepper.

3. In an extra-large skillet heat remaining 2 tablespoons olive oil over medium-high heat. Sear pork for 4 minutes on each side until golden brown. Transfer chops to a plate.

Add wine to skillet, scraping up any browned bits. Reduce pan juices for 1 minute.

4. Drizzle chops with pan juices before serving.

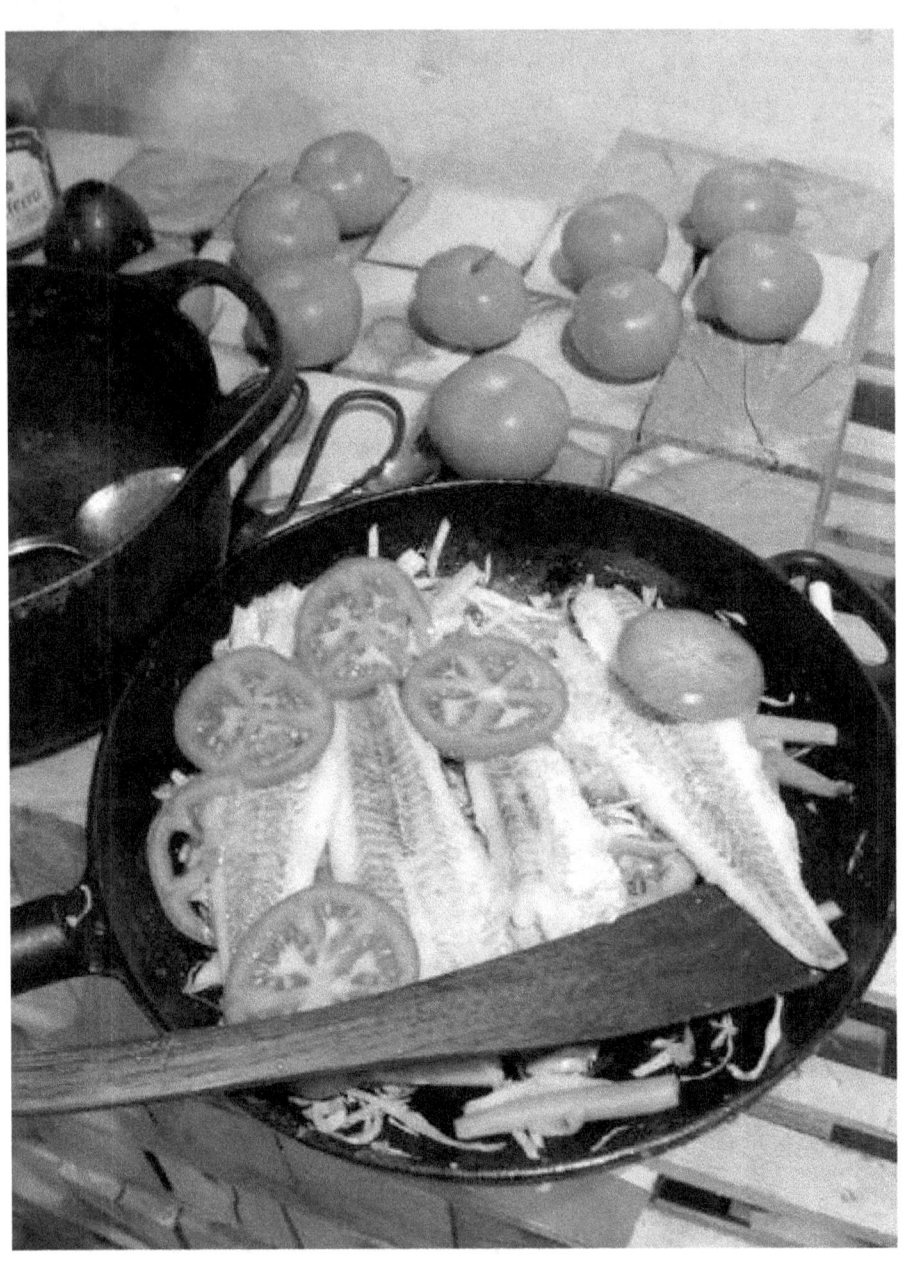

PORK CHOPS WITH A DIJON-PECAN CRUST

PREP: 15 minutes COOK: 6 minutes BAKE: 3 minutes MAKES: 4 servings PHOTO

THESE MUSTARD-AND-NUT-CRUSTED CHOPS COULDN'T BE SIMPLER TO MAKE—AND THE TASTE PAY-OFF FAR EXCEEDS THE EFFORT. TRY THEM WITH CINNAMON-ROASTED BUTTERNUT SQUASH (SEE RECIPE), NEO-CLASSIC WALDORF SALAD (SEE RECIPE), OR BRUSSELS SPROUTS AND APPLE SALAD (SEE RECIPE).

⅓ cup finely chopped pecans, toasted (see tip)
1 tablespoon snipped fresh sage
3 tablespoons olive oil
4 bone-in center-cut pork chops, about 1 inch thick (about 2 pounds total)
½ teaspoon black pepper
2 tablespoons olive oil
3 tablespoons Dijon-Style Mustard (see recipe)

1. Preheat oven to 400°F. In a small bowl combine pecans, sage, and 1 tablespoon of the olive oil.

2. Sprinkle pork chops with pepper. In a large ovenproof skillet heat the remaining 2 tablespoons olive oil over high heat. Add chops; cook about 6 minutes or until browned on both sides, turning once. Remove skillet from heat. Spread Dijon-Style Mustard on tops of chops; sprinkle with pecan mixture, lightly pressing into mustard.

3. Place skillet in oven. Bake for 3 to 4 minutes or until chops are done (145°F).

WALNUT-CRUSTED PORK WITH BLACKBERRY SPINACH SALAD

PREP: 30 minutes COOK: 4 minutes MAKES: 4 servings

PORK HAS A NATURALLY SWEET TASTE THAT PAIRS WELL WITH FRUIT. ALTHOUGH THE USUAL SUSPECTS ARE FALL FRUITS SUCH AS APPLES AND PEARS—OR STONE FRUITS SUCH AS PEACHES, PLUMS, AND APRICOTS—PORK IS ALSO DELICIOUS WITH BLACKBERRIES, WHICH HAVE A SWEET-TART, WINELIKE FLAVOR.

1⅔ cups blackberries

1 tablespoon plus 1½ teaspoons water

3 tablespoons walnut oil

1 tablespoon plus 1½ teaspoons white wine vinegar

2 eggs

¾ cup almond meal

⅓ cup finely chopped walnuts

1 tablespoon plus 1½ teaspoons Mediterranean Seasoning (see recipe)

4 pork cutlets or boneless pork loin chops (1 to 1½ pounds total)

6 cups fresh baby spinach leaves

½ cup torn fresh basil leaves

½ cup slivered red onion

½ cup chopped walnuts, toasted (see tip)

¼ cup refined coconut oil

1. For blackberry vinaigrette, in a small saucepan combine 1 cup of the blackberries and the water. Bring to boiling; reduce heat. Simmer, covered, for 4 to 5 minutes or just until berries are softened and color turns to a bright maroon, stirring occasionally. Remove from the heat; cool slightly. Pour undrained blackberries into a blender or

food processor; cover and blend or process until smooth. Using the back of a spoon, press pureed berries through a fine-mesh sieve; discard seeds and solids. In a medium bowl whisk together strained berries, walnut oil, and vinegar; set aside.

2. Line a large baking sheet with parchment paper; set aside. In a shallow dish lightly beat eggs well with a fork. In another shallow dish combine almond meal, the ⅓ cup finely chopped walnuts, and Mediterranean Seasoning. Dip pork cutlets, one at a time, in eggs and then in walnut mixture, turning to coat evenly. Place coated pork cutlets on a prepared baking sheet; set aside.

3. In a large bowl combine spinach and basil. Divide greens among four serving plates, arranging them along one side of the plates. Top with remaining ⅔ cup berries, the red onion, and the ½ cup toasted walnuts. Drizzle with blackberry vinaigrette.

4. In an extra-large skillet heat coconut oil over medium-high heat. Add pork cutlets to skillet; cook about 4 minutes or until done (145°F), turning once. Add pork cutlets to plates with salad.

PORK SCHNITZEL WITH SWEET-AND-SOUR RED CABBAGE

PREP: 20 minutes COOK: 45 minutes MAKES: 4 servings

IN THE "PALEO PRINCIPLES" SECTION OF THIS BOOK, ALMOND FLOUR (ALSO CALLED ALMOND MEAL) IS LISTED AS A NON-PALEO INGREDIENT—NOT BECAUSE ALMOND FLOUR IS INHERENTLY BAD, BUT BECAUSE IT IS FREQUENTLY USED TO CREATE ANALOGS OF WHEAT-FLOUR BROWNIES, CAKES, COOKIES, ETC., THAT SHOULD NOT BE A REGULAR PART OF A REAL PALEO DIET®. USED IN MODERATION AS COATING FOR A THIN SCALLOP OF PAN-FRIED PORK OR POULTRY, AS IT IS HERE, IS NOT A PROBLEM.

CABBAGE

- 2 tablespoons olive oil
- 1 cup chopped red onion
- 6 cups thinly sliced red cabbage (about ½ of a head)
- 2 Granny Smith apples, peeled, cored, and diced
- ¾ cup fresh orange juice
- 3 tablespoons cider vinegar
- ½ teaspoon caraway seeds
- ½ teaspoon celery seeds
- ½ teaspoon black pepper

PORK

- 4 boneless pork loin chops, cut ½ inch thick
- 2 cups almond flour
- 1 tablespoon dried lemon peel
- 2 teaspoons black pepper
- ¾ teaspoon ground allspice
- 1 large egg

¼ cup almond milk

3 tablespoons olive oil

Lemon wedges

1. For sweet-and-sour cabbage, in a 6-quart Dutch oven heat olive oil over medium-low heat. Add onion; cook for 6 to 8 minutes or until tender and lightly browned. Add cabbage; cook and stir for 6 to 8 minutes or until cabbage is crisp-tender. Add apples, orange juice, vinegar, caraway seeds, celery seeds, and ½ teaspoon pepper. Bring to boiling; reduce heat to low. Cover and cook for 30 minutes, stirring occasionally. Uncover and cook until liquid is reduced slightly.

2. Meanwhile, for pork, place chops between two sheets of plastic wrap or waxed paper. Using the flat side of a meat mallet or rolling pin, pound to about ¼ inch thickness; set aside.

3. In a shallow dish combine almond flour, dried lemon peel, 2 teaspoons pepper, and allspice. In another shallow dish whisk together the egg and almond milk. Lightly coat the pork cutlets in the seasoned flour, shaking off excess. Dip in the egg mixture, then again into the seasoned flour, shaking off excess. Repeat with remaining cutlets.

4. In a large skillet heat olive oil over medium-high heat. Add 2 cutlets to the pan. Cook for 6 to 8 minutes or until cutlets are golden brown and cooked through, turning once. Transfer cutlets to a warm platter. Repeat with remaining 2 cutlets.

5. Serve cutlets with cabbage and lemon wedges.

www.ingramcontent.com/pod-product-compliance
Lightning Source LLC
Chambersburg PA
CBHW071821080526
44589CB00012B/875